PAST-LIFE JOURNEYS
AND MESSAGES OF WISDOM

Past-Life Journeys and Messages of Wisdom

A Psychiatrist' s dramatic report on Human Soul

By Youngwoo Kim MD

ISBN: 9798615480720

CONTENTS

CHAPTER 1

Beginning Words

There seem to be two kinds of people in the world. The first one invest all their attention to the given premise of their daily lives, these are the ordinary people who generally adapt to various worldly problems without much thought or conflict. The second one, regardless of their occupation or what task they perform, are constantly irking themselves with questions like 'Who am I?' 'Where have I come from? and 'What is the true meaning and purpose of life?' The first group calls the latter 'immature dreamers' and the latter pity the former. But do these distinct types of people really exist? I do not wish to think so.

Deep inside, everyone must be questioning the origin and the meaning of his or her existence. As the answers are not easy to attain, most people live their lives pretending to have given up pursuing these answers. No one's life is free from the tastes of sorrow and frustration. No matter how successful or happy a person seems, he cannot escape the heart-breaking separation from loved ones or bitter frustration of unfulfilled wishes. Oppressed by this cruel destiny, we easily give up, get hurt, hurt one another to be defeated by our own lives. Who will help us to solve this problem? Where can we find true peace and comfort of mind? Will there be happiness at the end of life if we work to death to become rich and famous?

Will everything be OK, if we devote ourselves to religion? Some say that living one day at a time without thinking too much will do, but even such people will need a reasonable motive to go on like that. If the span of our existence is only 70-80 years before we return to absolute 'Nothingness', what value do the honesty and striving while alive would have?

In the eternal flow of time, our life span is only a fraction of a moment. Is it not fair and logical to enjoy this miserable short period of time to the fullest by any means? Why exert ourselves to anything when death will surely bring end to us all? What reason do we have to hesitate to harm and exploit others when everything will end in death? But, if we really have immortal souls in us, this question becomes very serious. And if our souls get rewards or punishments after death, according to the deeds we commit during life time, or we come back to earth in new bodies through reincarnation... Well, this might not be bad ideas to those who live honestly and seek the Truth. But to those who fear new and unfamiliar theory and prospect, this possibility will be burdensome and dreadful to accept. The brilliance and plenitude of materialism have added shine and abundance to people's lives, it has also misled us to judge the quality and meaning of people's lives - by the size of salary, cars and house we own.

Consciously or unconsciously, materialism commands our thoughts and emotions, lead us to the realm of materialism and traps us in the grinding wheel of endless competition. To have more, to climb higher, we push ourselves to exhaustion. In this busy world, who has time to contemplate on the existence of intangible and elusive soul? Overwhelmed by the work and toil to make ends meet, people bury existential questions deep in their bosoms.

But, frequent incidents of frustration, injustice, sorrow and despair in life stir up these deep-buried questions. 'Why do I fail after having done my best?' 'Why does such a nice person meet such a tragic fate?' 'Why do I suffer this terrible disease?' Agonizing moments in our life are numberless, and at the end of the questions raised by those painful events, the ultimate questions are bound to surface. 'Who am I, and where am I going to?' 'What is the meaning and purpose of my life?' 'What is the reason and meaning of my pain?'

These questions, that no one has answers to, frustrate us. Thus, in distress, we try to justify ourselves by spitting out bitter statements like

'Meaning of life is incomprehensible.' 'Life is a battlefield; we must seize whatever we desire.'

'Life is no big deal.'

This is my 14th year in the psychiatry, and is the 10th year since I became a specialist in psychiatry. So far, with my utmost, I have struggled to answer my own ultimate questions, as well as to understand and solve the symptoms and pains of my patients without much success. To my surprise, truly satisfying answers have visited me from unexpected direction in a mysterious form.

Those answers have illuminated my vague understanding of our souls and the world we live in, and they keep on providing me with the answers to my long-held questions. What you are about to read in this book are my unexpected encounters with mysterious beings and the messages from them.

The conversations in this book have not been altered at all from the taped recordings except for some unintelligible portions which may cause misunderstanding or confusion. The dialogues concerning my private life are largely omitted, but I swear upon my own career that no addition or distortion has been made to the transcription.

I feel there is a need to briefly review a few important issues to help readers to understand the contents of this book.

For the past 300 years, science has contributed tremendously to the improvement of human lives and civilization to earn the position of the highest worth. Armed with explainable and verifiable experiments and logics, science has been trying to solve the mysteries of Nature and Soul with the tools of physio-chemical laws. Many discoveries in Nature were possible since the Nature was phenomena of visible realm. However, as the human soul was invisible and untouchable, science has leaned toward denying its existence. Those who have witnessed the tremendous might of science became excited by the thought that this new power would resolve all of our problems. As the result, traditional value system of human society was shaken from its roots. The authority of religions and the respect toward mystery were replaced by new materialistic set of values. Yet, science has not been able to answer the questions, buried deep inside us, concerning the origin and the meaning of 'I'. Today, the danger of ill-used and abused science by immoral people has grown to threaten the very existence of mankind. The world is full of evidence of this grave threat. Severe and irreversible damages to nature and environments are going on all over the world in the name of industrial and economic development. So many species of insects, animals and trees are on the brink of extinction. People are being isolated in materialistic egoism and individualism; Powerful nations instigate wars between smaller countries for the growth of their war-related industry. Although abundance in goods is greater than ever, true peace and happiness are rare to be found. World is full of people who are suffering from steeper competition and higher than ever level of tension and anxiety. Will there be any chance that this flow of our society be turned around? Will it be impossible to leave a better world to our descendants?

Proving the existence of the soul has been a task which modern science could not achieve. By the same token, modern science has been powerless to disprove the existence of the soul. Concerning this metaphysical entity, current science is not much help. Various methods have been developed to prove the existence of the soul by many kinds of people during the last hundred years to encourage the emergence of a new field of study called 'Parapsychology.' So far, anecdotal evidences of claimed spiritual phenomena, photographs of human aura, second sight and clairvoyance have been reported. But we cannot yet tell what positive influence this evidence and study can exert upon our daily lives.

Apart from Parapsychology, for the last two decades, the research of Near Death Experience (NDE) has drawn much attention from scientists and lay people alike.

In my view, the common experiences reported by people who had NDE are very strong evidence of the existence of the soul, and a vital material in understanding the reality of death.

'What is the reality and essence of Death?' 'Is reincarnation Possible?' Major religions and folk-cultures around the world accept the existence of soul as indisputable fact. Since ancient times, various religions have taught the transmigration and reincarnation of human soul. In the early Judaism, as well as Buddhism and Hinduism, the transmigration of the soul was accepted as a truth.

Even Christianity had the doctrine of karma and transmigration, though emperor Constantine the Great of Rome and his mother, for political purposes, eradicated them in 355 AD from the New Testament. Also, in 553 AD, the teaching of transmigration was decided to be heresy in the Second Vatican Council again, this decision was probably a political scheme to control the public more effectively.

Belief in transmigration can be also found in ancient Egypt, Babylon, Assyria and Greece. Transmigration is a belief in which soul of human being undergo maturing process through long period of time and multiple and various forms of lives until it escapes from anguish and ignorance.

In this belief, people have been taught that death is nothing to fear, because it is only a passage to the world of souls, and to understand life, we must understand death also. The most important factor controlling transmigration is the law of Karma. - Karma is the sum of a person's actions in this and previous lives, viewed as a deciding power of the person's future existence. In a way, the concept of transmigration is a theory of soul evolution.

Recently, more intellectuals of the West, who are fed up and wearied with self-righteous philosophies and religion are seriously embracing the theory of transmigration because it is the most logical and reasonable theory to explain the countless contradictions and injustices of life. Furthermore, it is true that the researches in this field as well as the case studies of reincarnation are being conducted more seriously and enthusiastically in the Western world.

For more technical information regarding the cases of reincarnation and the theory of transmigration, I recommend the works of Ian Stevenson, MD. and Gina Cerminara, PhD. Ian Stevenson was a psychiatrist who researched cases of children who remembered their past-lives and wrote a book named 'Children Who Remember Their Past Lives'. The book presents many rigorously researched and verified cases of reincarnation that cannot be explained otherwise. Gina Cerminara has solved problems and healed symptoms of her clients through hypnosis and has conducted in-depth research on Edgar Cayce, one of the most famous clairvoyant of America. She also wrote 'Many Lives, Many Loves' and 'Many Mansions' combining theoretical explanations and case studies, and attracted much interest from the public.

WHAT IS HYPNOSIS?

The state of hypnosis means 'a state of increased suggestibility by focusing on one thought or phenomenon.' Simply put, it is a state of mind during which one can directly communicate with one's subconscious by temporarily bypassing the conscious mind. To elaborate on hypnosis, I may need more space than this one book offers. But it is important to know the brief history and background of hypnosis to read this book. Hypnosis has been used in all cultures since ancient times. It has been used in curing diseases and exorcising evil spirits by wizards and mediums as well as in ceremonies of various religions. In 1700s, Anton Mesmer, an Austrian medical doctor, without clear understanding of nature of hypnosis, attempted to use it to cure diseases as ancient healers might have done. He thought the hypnotic phenomena were caused by some form of Magnetism and called it 'Animal Magnetism.' Although the results of his attempt were promising in many cases and his popularity soared high in public, he soon found himself in a difficult position against backlashes and attacks by contemporary medical society. Consequently, the popularity and interest in hypnosis almost vanished from that time. Around mid 1800s, in England, came reports of various surgeries performed under influence of hypnosis as anesthesia. Near the end of 1800s, an English medical doctor named James Braid explained hypnosis in scientific view and used the term 'Hypnosis' for the first time. Afterwards, many French doctors, such as Jean Martin Charcot and Auguste Liebeault began serious research and practice of hypnosis. Hypnosis, once again, got attention and popularity from therapists and there came many important case reports and research results from them.

But with the introduction of Psychoanalysis by Sigmund Freud, hypnosis lost its shine and start to disappear from clinical practices.

It is believed that Sigmund Freud, who founded Psychoanalysis, was a student of Liebeaut and discovered the existence of subconscious part of human psyche through experiences in hypnosis. It is also rumored that

Freud turned to free association and psychoanalysis because he frequently failed in inducing hypnosis in his patients. In any event, hypnosis once again became forgotten as psychoanalysis gained popularity.

Since then, hypnosis has become a cheap trick of street and stage illusionists in exploiting people's curiosity to make money. This distorted and maligned image of hypnosis is still strong in public mind. But during the two World Wars, hypnosis was proved to be a very effective tool to treat shell-shocked and panicking soldiers, to attract attention of medical society. After the World Wars, extensive study of hypnosis began in 1950s, and in 1958, hypnosis was officially acknowledged by the United States Medical Association as a form of medical technique. In recent years, studies and applications of hypnosis in various clinical fields are dramatically increasing. I believe, in the future, hypnosis will be used for wider variety of patients than now.

Brian Weiss, an American psychiatrist whose book 'Many Lives, Many Masters' was recently published in Korea, claims in the book, that the memories of one's past lives can be recovered by time-regressing technique under hypnosis, and the causes of present problems can be found in these memories. The fact that one of the most elite intellectuals of a very reputable scientific profession wrote such a mysterious and incredible story might have come as a great shock to the general public. I have been using age-regression hypnosis to treat the traumas of childhood in some of my patients, and the ideas of transmigration and reincarnation of the soul sounded logical and worth researching to me, but was not paying much attention to them. But now, Brian Weiss's book suddenly came to me as a wake-up call to a new world to look into.

Modern psychiatry helps and treats many kinds of patients. As the images of mental clinic have improved much over the years, many patients voluntarily register and visit one to obtain treatment and medication. However, many are still visiting clinics secretively and reluctantly. Though there are individual differences, most patients improve with treatment to some degree.

But there also are patients whose symptoms don't improve and the causes of illness are hard to find. When a patient doesn't improve and the causes are elusive, it means only one simple truth, doctor's lack of knowledge to help the patient. But if doctors could not find the causes of the trouble even through the most advanced medical techniques as well as lengthy interview and analysis, they tend to blame the patients for their problems. Then, the patient, hurt and frustrated by the therapist's inability, embarks on his uncertain wandering search for a new therapist. As Medicine is an applied science with limited knowledge and abilities, it is impossible to explain all the patients with current theories and suppositions. Yet, are most doctors ready to accept new findings and explore new territories when their areas of specialty and familiar theories get challenged? Though it is a most proper duty for doctors to explore and evaluate the unfamiliar phenomena before dismissing them as mere illusions and mistakes, regrettably, such duty is not carried out often enough.

One day, late last summer, a female patient of mine with symptoms of mild depression recovered some memories of, presumably, a past life in a hypnosis session with me.

She had very vivid sight and feel of the past life. She saw an army general in his 40s in China around 800 AD. He was tall and stout in build, and was wearing magnificent body armor and leather boots of black color with gold patterns embroidered on them. He was sitting on a boulder overlooking other mountains and distant river branches shrouded in early morning mist, hardening his desperate resolution to fight the surrounding superior enemy force to his death.

The gold ornamental patterns on his clothes were so vivid to my patient's sight and the pang of his despair and resignation was so heart breaking that she broke into tears. A huge and curved sword on his side with an ornament attached to the handle also was clearly seen. At the moment of his death, an arrow, shot by the enemy, pierced him from back to chest. He sat and leaned against a column of a small pavilion on the mountain until his last breath. She recalled the burning and lingering pain after the arrow pierced him similar to electricity passing through from his back to the chest. A moment later, she saw him looking over his blood soaked dead body from above, there was no more pain, but comfort and relief. After the hypnosis session, the patient volunteered to draw the shape of the arrowhead and the patterns on the general's clothes in detail, and was shaken to the core by her own recollection. She could not dismiss the images of the scenery, people and the vivid realism of the tragic situation she saw and felt as hallucinations. She had never even dreamt or heard about such people and situation she saw in the recollection. And the instinctive realization that the general was herself, as well as her vivid and direct experience of his emotions was truly a wonder to her. She even remembered the general was called 'General Wu.' Beginning with this session, she recalled more memories of her various past lives in later sessions, and was healed of her life-long problems. Though there are many other interesting contents in her recollections, I must postpone the discussion of them for another time.

The editor in charge of 'Inner World Publishing Company' Kim Chul-Ho, was the man who translated 'Many Lives, Many Masters.' When I told him of my patient's past-life regression and my intention to research further into this field, he was very excited. He asked me if he may share this information with those who call him to ask further about the book and past-life regression therapy, I told him to do so. For the next several months, I selected some people who I believed needed hypnotic-regression therapy from both of my patients and those who called me out of curiosity. With them, I have had many age-regression and past-life regression sessions, and remarkable results started to accumulate.

The story you will read from now on is about mysterious experiences and messages that were given to one of my patient and me, by mysterious beings, in hypnosis sessions. In the messages, you may find some satisfying answers to the serious questions of your life. Though the story may sound mystical and incredible, when you read this book with your mind open, I am sure your attitude toward your life will change as much as mine did.

CHAPTER 2

The First Meeting:

The life of a Buddhist nun in Chosun Dynasty

(Chosun Dynasty 1392-1910: The last Dynasty in Korea established by
Yi Sung-Kye along with many progressive noblemen of the time.
Twenty seven Kings ruled over 519 years.)

One afternoon last autumn, I met a new male patient who made an appointment by phone call for a therapeutic interview. He was one of those who called me out of curiosity regarding Past-Life Regression Therapy. He was 26 years old college graduate, and was working for an average company. I saw goodwill and kindness in his face and he was a man of tall and large frame. His name was Won Jong-jin. As he sat facing me, he introduced himself with slight excitement and anticipation.

"Well. How shall I begin...? I have always been interested in many serious questions about life itself... I have read various books, and then I came across 'Many Lives, Many Masters' by Brian Weiss. The contents of the book really touched my heart. I have never done any meditation or self-training, but I have always been thinking, even while I work, that I want to become a clergyman someday... I go to church but not a true believer... Christianity rejects reincarnation, but I personally believe it exists. If we live more than one life time, we would have bigger chance of being saved. Wouldn't we? If we had lived where no Christianity was taught, we could be born again in the country of Christianity...I think it would be more reasonable... I don't have any particular problem, but I have a few things

I don't understand about myself. Sometimes I see a vision in my dream of what is going to happen, and things really happen as I saw in dream most of the time... My father died when I was twelve and now I live with my mother and a younger sister... I try to be nice to my sister but I can't stand her, because she always does hateful things. One more thing, other than I always dream of becoming a clergyman, I have always disliked China.

Whenever I think of the country, I feel afraid and abhorred, and I don't understand why. As I grow older, I dislike it even more. I am a little worried about this because I will have to go to China next year on a business trip...My mother have interfered with my life so much that there are many things I haven't been able to do until now. As she is a very self-sacrificing mother, I feel guilty when I should complain about her... and when I go to somewhere new, I often feel as if I had already been there before... At times, when I repress sexual impulse, I feel like I am a woman..." Besides this self-introduction, he told me about a few impressive dreams he has had.

I explained to him the fundamental principles and popular misconceptions of hypnotic regression and cautioned him not to expect too much from the first session. We moved to the therapy room and I had him laid half way on a reclining chair and made him to relax his tensions and guided him into the state of hypnosis. His reaction to my guidance was so good that I attempted to induce him to his past life right away. Followings are dialogue of the session.

K is I, and W is the patient Won.

K: Do you see anything around you?

W: (in a small and trembling voice)... It's a battle field... I am shaking with fear...

K: What are you doing there?

W: I am a woman... My name is Sun-rhe... I am twenty three years old... My clothes are all torn and soiled.

K: Tell me the things you see around you.

W: (in urgent and petrified voice)...Houses are on fire... it's desolate and dreary around... no dead bodies around...Two soldiers of Qing Dynasty are staring at me... destroyed houses are seen... I am afraid... I have a baby with me... I think I am going to be raped soon... (Breathing becomes raspy and starts to perspire heavily on his face)

(Qing Dynasty, 1636-1912: The last Dynasty of China, established by Nurhaci of Manchu, succeeding Ming Dynasty.)

K: Relax and leave the scene. We shall go to the next important scene...

W: (calm and steady voice)... It is a wedding ceremony...I am sixteen years old... I have no last name... and my husband's name is Park Chil-gap... He is seventeen years old... I borrowed and used someone else's last name...

K: Will you tell me what you see?

W: There are many relatives around... I am wearing bridal gown and head-piece... I am about 150 cm tall... and pretty... I don't think I wanted the marriage, but followed my parent's decision... My husband is tall, manly, trustworthy... but not handsome... he dies at thirty seven years of age...

K: What did you feel at the wedding ceremony?

W: I am happy...

K: Let's move to another scene.

W: After marrying him, my mother-in-law mistreated me much because I couldn't bear a child... but after two years, I had two daughters one after another... One of them died during the war... the dead one was whom I was holding at the battle field...

K: Where is the other one?

W: At home...

K: Will you move to another important event in that life?

W: ...I became a nun... In a Buddhist temple next to shoreline... I am a Buddhist priestess...

K: How old are you?

W: Twenty-seven...

K: Why did you become a nun?

W: After being raped by the soldiers of Qing Dynasty... village people called me 'whore' and... Eventually, I ended up leaving my home.

W: What is the name of the temple you are in?

K: It is made up of two characters... I see 'uh' which means 'fish' and ...I see big 'cho', the letter you can find on a Chinese Chess piece. (Since there is a Buddhist temple in Korea with similar name, I asked him later about it after the session, but he could not tell definitely if the name of the temple he saw was the same as the real one.)

K: What are your feelings there?

W: ...I try to forget my family... but it's not easy... I feel like I have given up everything... withdrawn and distressed.

K: What is your Buddhist name?

W: Yu-shim...

K: Let's move to your time of death...What do you see?

W: ...It is a small room in a monastery... I am lying down on the floor... There are three Buddhist nuns sitting around me.

K: How old are you?

W: Sixty-eight...

K: Did you suffer a disease?

W: Heart disease... a nun of about thirty years old and two younger nuns are present, and the oldest one is crying... (A little surprised voice)... The nun is one of my coworker in the company now... This is not an occasion to cry, but she does... (With calm voice)... I feel very comfortable...I am a very emaciated old woman...

K: Let's move to the moment of your death.

W: ... It is dark...Now it is bright again... I am floating in the room...I see my dead body, and the nuns are sobbing... I am now out of the room...

K: What do you see?

W: ...Blue sky... and a bright beam of light... I follow the light.

K: Following the light, tell me what you see.

W: I see what I should have done in that life... (In a remorseful voice)... I should have done more work; I could not help others much because I was broken down... The souls of the soldiers who raped me are so pitiful... (Dropping tears, his facial expression shows deep pain)... I should have taught myself more self-discipline and enlightenment, but I didn't do it properly... I could not ascend higher... (Became very emotional and started sobbing bitterly)

K: Please, calm down. Now we are moving back to the present...

I slowly woke him from hypnosis. After Won came to, he showed strong emotion of self-reproach and regret. Just before waking up from the trance he was in, he said that one of the daughters he saw is his present mother and those two soldiers who raped him are coworkers in his company. His expression after waking up was well worth seeing! He said that he felt delirious as if he had been hit on the head by a hammer, he could not completely believe what he saw and felt. We had a short discussion about the session and agreed to have another appointment. After he left with an expression of confusion and anguish on his face, I listened to the taped recording of the session and I felt sure that all the subtle and clear changes in his vocal tones and emotions were relevant to the situations he was in.

When the regression to one's past life succeeds for the first time, many enter directly into the most closely related event or situation of a particular life with the present problems. He was no exception. The reason for this is probably that the memory of such related events contains concentrated common emotional energies. Whether the memories recalled during past-life regression are genuine personal memories of the patient or mere fantasies is a controversial subject among academics. As a man of logical and scientific reasoning, I myself had such doubts also. But hallucinations or illusions of psychotic patients are never helpful in patient's recovery. When treating acutely psychotic patients, hallucinations usually are the first symptoms to disappear with medication. As psychotic hallucinations are incongruous and fragmented, contain contents of fearful, menacing nature, patients cannot describe their hallucinations as consistently as though they are watching an unfolding drama or a movie, as Won did. Those who realized the source of their present problems by exploring their past lives through regression usually experience dramatic improvement of their symptoms or problems. Similar, but less dramatic, improvements are seen in Psychoanalysis sessions, when a patient realizes certain connection between his current problems and the forgotten memories. As the patient understands the relationship between the two, the symptoms and sufferings take favorable turn. So, regression to one's past life can be seen only as an extension of currently used Hypno-Analytic age regression into the realm that lies prior to the moment of pregnancy.

The theory of Collective Unconsciousness, proposed by Carl Jung, suggests that certain groups of people possess a reservoir of memory, created by shared experiences and common cultural background, and the members of the group can access the memories in this reservoir. Though some scholars try to explain the past-life memories with this theory, the recovered memories from therapeutic regressions are very personal and vivid to defy this theory.

Furthermore, there are many cases in which the facts specified from those memories, such as who lived where at what time, were verified through serious researchers. And it is often that memories of one's past life reveal clues that help understand one's current personality traits, talent and weakness. Even in his first past-life experiences, Won recalled the scene which could be the cause of his vague fear and hatred toward China. He also realized that his present mother was the abandoned daughter in that life time, she came back with strong attachment and obsession on him to interfere with many things he wanted to do. The painful memory of being an abandoned child may be strong in her subconscious mind, making her to fear that he might abandon her again. Won also told me that he has been very interested in Buddhism itself, but felt very uncomfortable whenever he visited a Buddhist temple. As an unfortunate incident forced her to leave her family to lead the hard life of an ascetic priestess, the Buddhist temple not only served her as a shelter but also as a prison that constantly reminded her of her separation with her family. In his present workplace, he met those two soldiers and a priestess of the temple again, this may mean that Won still carries his share of Karma to resolve in his new relationships to them.

CHAPTER 3

The Second Meeting:

Life in Spain and India

Before starting the second session, Won and I exchanged some opinions regarding the previous session. He told me briefly of his thoughts.

"It was quite marvelous... as I think of it, I find that I detest especially the Qing Dynasty the most in the history of China... and the fact that I was a woman may explain how I feel womanish when I try to repress my sexual urges. But, all of this could be a work of imagination; I made up all in my head... I am not sure yet... I still don't know what is what... Then, again, if it were true, my interest in religious occupation and the seeking of the Truth can be explained well enough..."

After moving to the therapy room, we started the second session and soon found ourselves in the 14th century, Spain.

K: Will you tell me what you see?

W: ...I see a fortress wall... It looks very old...I am a soldier... Actually, I was a farmer but was drafted because of war...

K: Can you tell me about your clothes and appearances?

W: ...I am wearing a metal helmet... and have armor on my chest... but my shoes are shabby and cheaply made...

K: Your name and age?

W: ...I am twenty three years old... Jose Martinez is my name... I am very afraid and anxious now... (in a trembling voice, suppressing agitation)... I am only an ordinary farmer, but I have to fight in a war...

K: What is the year?

W: ...I see numbers in front of my eyes...1, 3, 3, 8 ...I think it is the year 1338.

K: What is the name of the place?

W: ...Castile... It is a castle in Castile...

K: Who are the enemies in the war?

W: It is war against Islam...

K: Do you know the name of your commander?

W: …Miguel.

K: Is he a general?

W: ...He is a Knight under the Lord of Castile...

K: Let's move to another scene... to when you were very young... What do you see?

W: I am five years old ...I am playing with my friends... and a friar just passed by us... we bowed to him...

K: Who is the friar?

W: He is friar Mitchell... he is a fat one...

K: Can you tell me about your family?

W: ...I have parents, one younger brother and one younger sister...

K: Do you know your mother's name?

W: ...Maria Garta... My younger sister is Sophia...

K: Let's move to a scene where your family gathers.

W: ...We are eating... Father sits across from me, he is a farmer... He is a massive man with plenty of beard...

K: Will you tell me about your house and other things around you?

W: ...It is a very poor farmhouse... ordinary home, very shabby... A light is on and we are sitting on rough wooden benches... We are eating some food boiled... simmered dish ... no other food do we have...

K: Tell me about your mother.

W: She is quiet and don't speak much... but the atmosphere in the house is happy one...

K: Let's move to another scene.

W: ...I am sitting in a forest... I can see the fortress wall... I am sixteen years old... I am sitting there with a girl I like very much...

K: Is it a friend from the village?

W: Yes... Her name is Anna, thirteen years old...

K: What do you feel there?

W: ...I am happy...

K: What are you two talking about?

W: ...Just trivial things and ordinary matters... Anna likes me too...

K: Let's move to another moment.

W: (Desperate and hushed voice)... In the last battle, I had my one leg cut off... just above the knee by a sword...

K: Do you feel pain?

W: No I don't...

K: What was the result of the war?

W: We won...but I don't understand why we must have such wars...

K: Move to another event.

W: ... I am in a Cathedral ... It is in the middle of a Mass... There are many people in the cathedral.

K: Can you tell me what you see in the cathedral?

W: ... The nobles sit in the front, and we peasants sit in the back. I am sixteen years old... I am not focusing on the Mass ceremony ...Anna and I are looking at each other furtively... adults don't know that. There is an aisle in the middle; I am sitting on the right and Anna on the left, one row behind...

K: What is your feeling at this time?

W: (with a joyous expression)... Delightful!

K: Next scene... please.

W: ...I have a wooden leg and I am farming...

K: Do you have family?

W: ...I have one daughter and wife...

K: Is your wife Anna?

W: ... I am not sure...

K: Can you see her closely?

W: ..... She is not the one I loved...

K: What is your wife's name?

W: Martha...

K: How old are you at this time?

W: Thirty-six

K: Are you happy?

W: No

K: Why didn't Anna and you marry?

W: ...I married according to my parents' decision... Anna did not get married... She became a maid in the Lord's mansion...

K: Was Anna pretty?

W: (sadly)...She was beautiful to me... But she wasn't the most beautiful woman.

K: When did you two get separated?

W: When I was twenty-five.

K: Was it because you lost a leg?

W: ...No it's not... The Lord was too powerful... since Anna's family was too poor; they had to send Anna as a maid.

K: How did you meet your wife?

W: ...She was a wandering Gypsy... She settled down and lived with me...

K: How did you feel about the loss of one leg?

W: ... I gave up on it... But losing a leg did not become a big handicap...

K: Were you mentally impoverished as well by the war?

W: No...

K: What was the most difficult thing in that life?

W: ...I was a very considerate man... I had little greed and sought for a serious and solemn life, I was taciturn since I learned only little... but I lived my life, thinking deeply about the most important thing.

K: What is the most important thing?

W: To help others to become better...

K: Were your parents still alive at this time?

W: Both of them passed away by then...and my younger sister was married off to a faraway place...

K: What is the name of your village?

W: ... I lived there... without moving anywhere... Minon, it is called something like that.

K: Let's move to another scene.

W: ...I think I am about to die now...

K: How old are you?

W: ...Fifty-four

K: Why are you dying?

W: ...My bowels are not well... I have been that way for my whole life...

K: Who's around you?

W: My wife...

K: Do you love her?

W: Yes... I thought about Anna a lot, but I love my wife...

K: Where is your daughter?

W: I don't' see her now... but, having not married, she lives with us.

K: Shall we move to the moment of death?

W: (After repeating deep breathing several times, he recovered composure again)... I see an angel... I just died... The angel is waiting for me...

K: Is the angel familiar to you?

W: No...

K: Will you tell me what you see?

W: ...I am still in the room... my wife is weeping, muffling her cry...

K: What do you feel?

W: ... I feel sympathy toward my wife and I have much expectation for the next life to come...

K: Did you expect the next-life while you were alive?

W: No...

K: Are you feeling free?

W: Yes... but I am not completely free... It's because of the things I cannot carry with me...

K: What are they?

W: I didn't enjoy true peace...

K: Was 'true peace' your task of the life?

W: ...Someone is talking to me... he tells me to possess the true peace...

K: Where are you now?

W: ...I am flying the sky...

K: Tell me more of that life.

W: ...I lived without being able to express my own opinion, not even once... I had always been a man of obedience...While young, I obeyed my lord, I lived obeying the fate as I grew old... but I had no peace... it wasn't despair, though... I learned something in this life... it is that this was the last of my materialistic lives... From then on, spiritual lives would unfold... This life was a turning point...

K: How do you know that?

W: I hear a voice right next to me... I hear a voice and it is transmitted to my mind as well... After this life, I evolved mentally and spiritually...

K: Was it a leap of one level?

W: (solemnly)...Two levels... It was a crucial life... I don't hear the voice anymore...

K: Rest a while, and wake up slowly...

The second life was in Spain. One of the important questions in transmigration is whether we repeat reincarnation only within our own culture or country of birth. In my experiences of past-life regression with many people, the reincarnation into the same region or culture was not a law. Of course, even souls may have tendencies to be attracted to familiar backgrounds. According to Francis Story, a researcher of transmigration, 'There are more cases of one being reincarnated at, or near the place one died, provided that the conditions remain similar.' Though I generally agree to his opinion, yet, I think it's more reasonable to accept that our souls need to encounter and experience many different cultures and situations in many different lives in various countries to evolve and grow.

Having the memory of a life on the other side of the earth suggests that the memories of past-lives are not recorded in our hereditary genes. Since no ancestors could have moved from one continent to another in each generation, they could not possibly have mixed with the genes of other human races.

If the memories of each past life are from the different cultures, the theory of Collective Unconsciousness of a tribe falls short in explaining the phenomenon.

The most simple and logical conclusion should be that the memories are the results of direct experiences during different life times of the individual.

Why is it so difficult to accept the idea of transmigration? Because it is unfamiliar and offending to our material oriented mentality. To be accountable for our own actions according to the law of Karma would be a noble and just idea that will make us to live with more consideration and responsibility toward others. But, for those who wish to escape from responsibilities and consequences of their actions, the theory of reincarnation would be a big discomfort. Once we accept the possibility of reincarnation, the way we view our life would change. Being able to see the purpose and direction of our life, we would become to appreciate it wholeheartedly. Whether to accept or reject something, we need to know about it. Thus the science should work to find answers to the question of reincarnation and transmigration. Dismissing the memories of past-life as mere fantasy is very unscientific attitude, accumulating reports of past-life regression and healed symptoms and illness through the therapy are too many to ignore.

The life of poor and disabled 'Jose', who lost a leg in war and parted from the loved one, must have forced Jose to turn to introspection and to seek inner peace to endure and survive the agonizing reality. When he lost Anna, he must have felt as if he would perish under the pain of the loss, yet, his life pulled his existence forward with its unyielding tenacity. I think many of us are no stranger to such loss and misery. Even with each foot on the realms of life and death, contemplating to end all in suicide, we eventually pull ourselves through the loss and survive. Overcoming despair and self-denial through losses and frustrations of our life, we grow to mature and understand the pain of others. When alive, Jose was a Catholic, the religion of the area at the time. Surely, the idea of reincarnation must have been unthinkable to him at the time and the environment, but he immediately realized that there was another life waiting for him after his death. This, I believe, is due to the recovery of his innate Self and its knowledge of transmigration as his soul shed its physical body.

According to the Near-Death-Experience testimonies, what we experience after death depends largely on the experience and cultural background of the deceased. The main reason for this might be that the domain of souls is of metaphysical sort, in which our imaginations about after-death-world while alive become realized after our actual death. Another reason could be to lighten the soul of the shock of suddenly changed environment after death by providing familiar settings. What Jose heard could have been the voice of a so called guiding-angel.

Jose's learning that his life was 'the last stage of materialistic life' supports the theory of transmigration that our souls learn and develop through reincarnation.

Though his life time was spent in poverty and despair of losses, his soul made significant growth. After waking up, Won said that the wife in Jose's life was the woman he almost married in this life, and Jose's parents are his parents in this life. The mother's personality is little bit different but the father's stayed the same. The mother in Jose's life was the daughter in Sun-rhe's life, and again, Won's mother in his present life. The experience of death in past-life regression is very important. The pain and cause of the death can be changed into powerful thought energy field and etched into the soul's memory to resurface as unexplained fear or anxiety in the future lives. If a patient's symptoms arise from such a cause, no amount of common psychotherapy would be helpful. There are plenty of cases in which the memories of death from past lives turn into phobias in this life. For some example, those who drowned would fear swimming pools, those who died of hunger and exhaustion in a cave would compulsively avoid dark and confined places and who had fallen from a cliff can show acrophobia and so on. Though it would be a folly to see all phobias in this view, certain phobias that cannot be resolved by various treatments and analysis may have their roots in the trauma of past lives. Jose did not feel the pain on his severed leg, maybe because Won looked at it as if he were watching a movie, separated from the scene. However, there are many patients who feel severe pain vividly when they re-live painful situation in the past lives. In such cases, the therapist must be able to help the patient to relieve the pain and reassure the patient that everything is okay before continuing the session.

After a brief rest, we departed again to search for his third life.

K: Where are you now?

W: ...It is the 15th Century now... I am a beggar in India... My age is forty-nine...

I am a beggar, but I am not embarrassed... It's because I know what others don't...

K: Can you tell me of your appearances?

W: ...I am very gaunt and ...my clothes are tattered... but my eyes are sparkling...

K: Do you have family?

W: No, I don't... I left my home when I was young... I used to live among extended family... They were of noble status...

K: What is your name?

W: ...Shantagra... or similar to that... I am from Bengal...

K: Tell me about your parents.

W: My family was one of the most powerful clan in the region... My father had immense political power...I left home because I hated my father's bureaucratic trickery... He wanted to marry me off for his political gain, but I refused him...

K: What is your father's name?

W: ...It starts with the sound 'Gal'...

K: How old were you when you left home?

W: ...I was twenty five... I was not married yet, and there were my mother and many relatives in the house... the house always teemed with people... and I had many step-brothers as well.

K: What did the house look like?

W: ...The house shows tremendous amount of wealth and extravagance...

K: Why did you leave?

W: ...I was not the son who satisfied my father... My father had wanted to pass his power to me, though...

K: Were your personalities much different?

W: If I were to follow his steps... I had to kill people... I was not for such things... I loved poems and flowers...

K: Can you tell me about your brothers?

W: ...One of my younger brothers had his eyes on my position...

K: What was his name?

W: ...Samanta... his name was Samanta.

K: What is the year?

W: It's...mid 15th Century.

K: Can you tell me about the society you lived in?

W: ...Rich people enjoyed immeasurable wealth... and the poor suffered their poverty severely... I was not interested in the society itself, I was absorbed in my ascetic practices...

K: Have you been a beggar since you left home?

W: Correct...

K: What did you do for yourself for discipline and asceticism?

W: ...I sought and met enlightened sages in Himalayas, and learned from many teachers...

K: Let's move to another scene...

W: (Suddenly his voice changed - very low pitch and solemn it became)

...There are certain parts in my ascetic practice that I am not content with... because it is only for the benefit of me... My practice was not any help to others... My past lives did not bring peace to me in this life... Instead, at present, the religion and the asceticism I practice bound my soul... the real Truth is not in self-contentedness, but it is in providing benefits to many by sharing my life...

K: Do you hear the voice that spoke to you before?

W: ...The voice comes from outside...

K: Where are you now?

W: ...I am looking at the beggar... I am over sixty years old now...

K: Is the voice talking about the beggar?

W: No... (a little surprised)...someone is instructing me now...

K: Listen to it, please.

W: (In a deep and vibrant and solemn voice)... Many people seek contentment through religion, but it only bounds them and makes people around them to suffer... The goal of the search for the real Truth depends on how many people improve together, and purify their souls through the process... Ascetic practice that does not purify one's soul is like glittering cheap ornaments on oneself, and is not different from what wealthy woman decorates herself with things of vanity... What is more dangerous is that those with worldly vanity can be taught of its folly, but to those with vanity of the soul, no one can teach the Truth... Hence, they die without even knowing their soul's impoverishment... yet, no one realizes that he decays from inside... The correct road to true asceticism is to help and serve others, through one's realization of innate Self, so that they can walk their way of life... The most important aspect in ascetic practice is sacrifice... Perfection of the Truth is love...and the prerequisite of love is sacrifice... Practice sacrifice ...Sacrifice can appear as transgression and heresy to the eyes of the others... It may appear in a totally unexpected form as well... but practice sacrifice... Only after the sacrifice, true love can come... Only those who practice love are the ones who have mastered the Truth... All other efforts practiced without this understanding, is like an echo in an empty space...because there is no fruit to it... This man's life (Won seemed to be pointing to himself by nodding slightly) will turn out the same... He has repeated many days in many lives, yet he still is confined in the loop without understanding... it is because he is feeble in truly serving others... he has not practiced enough... (after pausing awhile)... Sacrifice must be practiced... When it is done, our souls will become freer than before...(returning to Won's voice) ... The voice stops here.

K: Do you see anything?

W: I can't see myself.

K: Relax and rest awhile...

When I woke him after a short rest, he told me about the voice he heard in hypnosis. 'The voice was very clear and the meaning of the message was transmitted to my heart as well... I may call it a telepathy, depending on what it said, I received strong feelings and visual images as well... The voice was very soft, smooth and friendly, but deep and weighty too... I felt a being or beings, spiritually much higher than me, were instructing me...' An auditory hallucination does not occur like this, it usually comes with fragmentary, irrelevant, incoherent and negative contents, and many of the contents are derogatory and destructive.

But this voice, as an empathic and logical observer, described the situation Won was in and elucidated the teachings within it. This is the same nature as that of the 'Master' which Brian Weiss described in his book. Since 'Master' is not familiar word to Koreans, and there is not even a close word to designate it in modern Korean language, I would like to refer the voice as 'Voice of the Wise' or simply 'the Voice.' In whatever name they are called, I believe they are transcendental, higher spiritual beings than us. I believe the voices of angels described in the Bible are probably from the same kind. They can be understood as beings that lead and assist the growth of human souls through the wisdom of their already advanced status. What we often call as guardian angels or Spirits may also be these beings. Won's life in India was a sincere one, but the Voice said that the life of ascetic practice and self-realization is not enough. The claim that ascetic practice and effort for oneself alone yields no fruit but emptiness is not any different from the statement 'Saving the Mass' in Mahayana Buddhism or 'Love thy neighbors' in Christianity. We might suspect Won fabricated the part of the Voice which praised 'Love', as he is a Christian in his present life. However, the statement which instructs 'self-sacrifice' without being tied to certain religion or religious teachings even though it may appear to be transgression and heresy is not a usual teaching of Christian Churches. As Won said, his life in the 14th Century Spain was the last materialistic one, the life in India, in which he left his family to seek spiritual practice, could have been his next one. However, his soul was not able to advance much, since he failed to overcome the limit of selfish ascetic life. He realized this only after he ended that life. This would be another evidence of transmigration of the soul – The duty of the soul is to learn and mature from its mistakes in successive lives. Religions of today teach people not only good things but also bad parts that are contaminated by human arrogance and prejudice. If some people believed everybody else, except those in their own sect of religion, is going to hell and that is what justice is about, then they are not truly religious people but factionists and severe egotists. The reason that more people are getting frustrated by religions of today and seek for something new is because they often see contradictions and shades of falsehood in the real lives of religious people, instead of love and truth seeking. The Voice referred to these styles of faith as 'glittering ornaments.' and claimed that the true religion is self-sacrifice, servitude and love to help others grow.

CHAPTER 4

The Third Meeting:

Lives and Realizations in Chosun, Koguryo and Scotland

A week after the second regression, we sat facing each other again. He told me what he had been contemplating about during the last week. "I think I am learning a lot from Past-Life Regression sessions... I now think, the way how I live is the most important, social status and wealth mean nothing... Focusing on what I should do in the present life is the most important thing... In my current religious life, I should become more assertive and active, take initiative and go forward... If the people in my church knew that I believe in reincarnation, they will try to dissuade me. But, someday they will understand... It seems to me that the souls of people have differences in quality... there are rich and famous people with immature or barren souls, and there are almost invisible people with more advanced souls... I did some research on the history and geography of Spain, and I found a region called Castile. I hadn't known the name before the research because I have never been interested in geography..."

The confused and incredulous expression on his face and uneasy attitude he showed after the last regression therapy had totally disappeared and I could sense a subtle but positive change in him. In this session, I decided to follow wherever his subconscious mind leads us.

The fourth life was in Chosun Dynasty, Korea

K: Where are you now?

W: ...Next to a creek

K: Are you alone?

W: I am doing my laundry... There are other women, too

K: What is your name?

W: ...I am called Gobdani (means Pretty Girl)...

K: What is the year?

W: ... It is 1631... I am sure of it.

K: What is the season?

W: ...It is turning from spring to summer...

K: How are your feelings?

W: ...Not bad... I feel pretty good, actually... I am washing clothes without much thought.

K: Let's move to an important event of the life...

W: ...I married to a male servant in the house when I was eighteen...

K: Are you a servant as well?

W: Yes...

K: How is your appearance?

W: ...Pretty, good looking...

K: Where do your parents live?

W: ...As we are servants tied to the house over the generations, my parents live in the same house...

K: What is the name of your husband? W: He is called... Dolsoe

K: Let's go forward to the next important event... Do you see anything?

W: ...An old woman... Sixty-two years old...

K: Don't you see other people?

W: There are my son and his wife...two grand children. Our master granted us a piece of land to support ourselves... We are farming in that land... The master passed away when my husband was forty-four years old...

K: What region is it?

W: ...Kyungsang Province (Southeast part of Korea)

K: Where in that province?

W: Hapchun or Uiryong... I am not sure...

K: Is this life peaceful and ordinary?

W: (As if he was waiting for the question, the answer came immediately)... This is a resting life...

K: To rest is the purpose of this life?

W: Yes...

K: Was there no hardship at all in the life?

W: ...The work was not too hard... very ordinary life...

K: Move to the moment of your death...

W: (with a tense expression)... Sixty-three... I died by falling from a high place...

K: Why did you fall?

W: ...I slipped my footing...

K: What were you doing before you fell?

W: ...I was picking edible herbs in a mountain...

K: Were you healthy?

W: Yes... I see my funeral procession... I am in the white hearse... They are burying me on a small slope... My family members are in deep sorrow...

K: Where are you now?

W: ...I don't know...

K: Relax and rest...

A life to rest.

It is interesting to know that there is such a life, peaceful and comfortable without big conflicts or misfortunes. Like a blessed vacation between two long and hard semesters in school, a life of rest and peace between two difficult lives could be a merciful consideration from God. To our eyes, her unexpected sudden death at the end of her comfortable life may seem to be a big misfortune. However, in a larger perspective, it may not necessarily be so to herself. She was born into the house of a generous master, gained his trust enough to earn her own house and a piece of land. Won said later on "She lived her life not as a slave, but almost as a free self-sufficient person and I felt that sudden and tragic accidents around us are not without higher reasons."

In fact, modern medical science has little knowledge regarding death. Though there may be a definition of bodily death, I don't remember learning anything about the meaning of death itself during both of my medical school days and the training years of residency to become a psychiatrist. Does physical death mean expiration of my 'Self?' Medicine today is reluctant to discuss this question. Considering the fact that the basis of modern medical science is the materialistic world view, this reluctance to deal with any metaphysical question seems natural to me.

However, for those who lost their loved ones and friends to death, it would be unacceptable and hard to understand that such vivacious and vibrant lives just disappeared into eternal nothingness in one instant. If those loved ones, who shared happiness and endured frustrations together are nothing but waste of efforts and patience, why should we value this momentary life?

If the death is the end of the 'Self', life itself must be a meaningless flicker on a passing moment.

Religion and philosophy ponder on death. Religions have their own views and teachings on the subject but these are the products of influence and distortion by the overall scheme of each religion, and can be totally different from knowing the actual substance of death objectively.

Philosophy also can provide no better explanation than religions'.

Any philosopher's rambling about the concept of death in complicated terms and wordplay is only a bluff to cover his ignorance. If we truly wish to understand death, we'd better study ancient scriptures and modern documents about it. Ancient people studied and understood death because it was so common all around them. They had to deal with death in everyday life to endure and bear the unbearable losses of loved ones. I believe all the meditations and ascetic practices were born in this abundance of sorrow and despair in ancient people. Through these techniques, they overcame the sorrows of life and realized the existence of eternal Soul. Among many ancient texts regarding death, 'The Tibetan book of the Dead' contains outstanding and specific contents. It emphasized that we must face death in peaceful state of consciousness. Egyptians, Greeks and Romans all had well developed understanding of death and mysterious experiences, but none of their books described the process of death as this one did.

The Bhagavad Gita, an ancient Indian scripture describes the principle of reaching the next life after passing death: 'According to the last things one thinks at one's death, next life is decided. In other words, 'one attains what one's mind is focused on.' In another Indian scripture 'Upanishad', it is stated that 'Those who don't reach realization will repeat death eternally.' Both explain the concept of Karma and Transmigration. Teaching of Buddha on this is the same.

Buddhist scriptures instruct that you cannot break the bind of your 'Self' without realization, thus you never escape the endless transmigration.

Although there are slight differences, all ancient cultures accepted the ideas of life after death, judgment, the after-world and reincarnation. Many people today may dismiss such teachings as outdated superstition and allegory, if not laughable jokes. But, when we look into such ancient teachings closely, we can find many answers to the basic questions of life. They contain the valuable teachings of realization on how we could reach true oneness by overcoming the limit of sectarian religions.

Won said that his images in the past lives appear to him in mixed form of still photos and movie-like clips. He also said that the explanation of a scene appeared in written words and the messages were transmitted into his head along with images to help him understand what he saw.

Sometimes he actually re-lived the scene himself within the screen projected into his head and sometimes he watched them from the third person point of view like watching a movie.

His Fifth life was in Koguryo Dynasty in 623 AD (Koguryo Dynasty: BC ?-AD 668: An ancient dynasty in Korea, famous for its people's energetic spirits and excellent horsemanship. Koguryo fought for the hegemony of Eastern Asia against China for more than 700 years during the Three Kingdom Period. The Kingdom spread on the northern part of Korea as well as Manchuria and the north region of Great Wall, China)

K: Can you tell me what you see?

W: ...I see horses... This is Koguryo in 623 AD.

K: What do you look like? What are you doing?

W: ... I am a young man of about twenty years of age... I am one of noble men in the kingdom... I am returning home after horse riding and hunting...

K: What is your name?

W: Kulgulji...

K: Are you alone?

W: I am with a friend... his name is Mulhulnewu

K: Is his name four syllable words?

W: Yes.

K: Where are you?

W: ...In the province of north... I see a dense forest here...

K: What is the season?

W: ... Late spring...

K: Are there others around you?

W: There are some of my servants...

K: What game did you catch in the hunting?

W: I did not hunt much... Two rabbits I caught... The hunting itself was not the purpose of this expedition... The real purpose was to talk and spend time with my friend...

K: Do you have any title or official job?

W: ...I will soon be appointed to a government post... My father is a high official...

K: Your father's name?

W: Kulshibuzung...

K: Is it a title?

W: His name.

K: Do you have siblings?

W: ...I have three brothers and one younger sister...I am the second-born.

K: How is the political situation of your country?

W: Not very good...I have been talking about matters of state with my friend...the royal authority has weakened...bureaucrats now rule the country...There are suspicious movements in China and new powers rising in the Tang Dynasty...and the relationship with warlords near the border have become quite worrisome. The morale of Koguryo is crumbling and our high spirits of defending the fatherland with strong military power is no longer valued much...Noblemen are only obsessed with their worldly gain... The news about a lord in Yodong region who committed many immoral deeds to satisfy his greed has become a very popular topic of conversation...

(Tang Dynasty period in China : AD 618-AD 906, Yodong region: Eastern part of Yo river in northeastern part of China.)

K: What is the name of the lord?

G: Galchiger...

K: Let's move to a scene where all your family members are gathered... What are they doing?

W: ...Dining...mother and all family members are gathered...

K: How is your father dressed?

W: He changed into comfortable clothes which he often wears in the house... he is talking to us about what happened in the Royal Court today... Mother is well disciplined person with good spirits... she is very obedient to my father... my older brother has married... we are getting along quite well...

K: Can you describe your clothes?

W: ...It is made of silk... it looks somewhat like Taekwondo uniform...

K: Does it look like the Koguryo clothing in ancient Korean tomb painting?

W: Yes...exactly the same...

K: What's on the dining table?

W: There are many kinds of green herbs... and a chicken dish too... I see different cookies and... very fragrant alcoholic drink... and I don't know the names of many other dishes... many servants are serving... It's a big household...

K: Will you tell me the shape and structure of the house?

W: ...It is different from the traditional Korean houses I used to see... We have our own soldiers in the house... about three hundred of them we have... the courtyard is vast...but lodgings for people are not as spacious...

K: Does your household manage all three hundred private soldiers?

W: Yes... they belong to my father... They are loyal only to him...

K: Is your father's rank very high among noblemen?

W: He is responsible for a very important function, but he does not have much real power...His function is almost like that of the Minister of Interior... (in a sudden, bitter voice)... I think my father is being purged...Yes, he is purged...

K: Why is he purged?

W: He is resented by Yeonkaisomun...

(Yeonkaisomun: A warlord who wielded immense power near the end of the Koguryo period. He resisted the China friendly political atmosphere of the time and appointed his own king to concentrate scattered political powers. He saved Koguryo from the invasion of Tang forces.)

K: What is the title of Yeonkaisomun?

W: ...He is not prominent now... but he will seize the power in time... My father is of higher rank at present though.

K: Let's go forward in time.

W: ...(bitterly) My family is totally ruined... I am stabbed...perhaps dead...I can see myself lying on the courtyard...

K: How old are you?

W: ...Nearly forty years old...

K: Were you still living with your family then?

W: Yes, we all lived together... I have two sons...

K: Did someone attack your family?

W: One of Yeonkaisomun's subordinate did...one of his staff officers...

K: Do you know his name?

W: ...Makhoji or a similar name

K: What year is it?

W: Maybe 648... it is before 650.

K: All of your family died?

W: Yes... we all died... Only my younger sister survived since she lived away after marriage... my parents and brothers all died and the soldiers of my house are either dead or scattered...

K: Why did they kill you?

W: Yeonkaisomun tried to build up his power and my father was opposing him... They were not exactly political rivals...but each belonged to the opposite side... My father was revered by me... I respected my father...

K: How did you die?

W: I was stabbed from behind...

K: What was the title of your post in the government? W: ...Dairiji...

K: What do you do?

W: ...My job is similar to those of today's Ministry of Government Administration and Treasury combined... it is not a high post... a middle one...

K: Is your wife dead too? W: Yes...

K: What was like the territory of Koguryo at that time?

W: ...It occupied much of the Asian Continent on the Chinese side...Certain clans near our border, such as Malgal, were difficult to manage, so we didn't conquer them... But their areas were virtually our land anyway...Our power reached farther than that of Tang Dynasty... We were smaller in territory but the power of our territory was much stronger than that of Tang Dynasty... And we were very confident in managing the territory too (the voice was very proud and resolute in tone).

K: What were the things you had to do in that life?

W: ...Not to be obsessed with possession... I had to learn that things like political status and affluence are not big help in attaining happiness... I didn't have much greed though... being revered in society did not have much meaning...

K: What do you feel about being attacked like that?

W: I feel, I have been expecting such an attack for a long time...

K: Have you been anxious always?

W: Yes...I have been nervous from long ago...

K: We are leaving that life... Please relax and rest...

In the long history of Korea, not much record or items of Koguryo remain now. Hardly any record of the kingdom was preserved because Shilla – one of the Three Kingdoms – eventually unified Korea after defeating Koguryo. So the historians of Shilla deleted and distorted all the glorious and remarkable achievements of Koguryo from history books. Most of the remaining ancient histories of Korea were written by historians who were born long after the Three Kingdom period. Although no historian would acknowledge the memories attained through Past-Life-Regression as objective evidence, we have had a glimpse of an ancient nobleman's life through Won's recollections. The fact that each of the noble household was to own hundreds of private soldiers shows us how they would have wielded such strong military might against rivals and enemies alike according to the political situations.

Won recalled the territory of Koguryo ran deeply into the mainland China, and its powerful influence reached farther than that of Tang Dynasty. This corresponds to the claims of progressive Korean historians. Won explained after waking up from hypnosis that the land of the Warlords' of

Koguryo spread from the north of Tang to the western frontiers of China forming a long strip of defense line to check the power of Tang from spilling over. Won also said "The policy of respecting more powerful countries and receiving tributes from weaker countries and the policy of suppressing one barbaric nation by another one, were what Tang learned from Koguryo." He also said that the actual military and political situation at the time was that Koguryo was slightly pressing Tang Dynasty, and Koguryo did not abuse peoples of conquered nations as slaves like Sparta of ancient Greece did although its population was rather small for its larger power spheres.

When talking about the territory and the power of his nation, Won sounded like an enthusiastic patriot who boasts about his country. His voice was strong and full of pride. Whether what he said was completely true or not, at that moment, he transformed into a proud nobleman of Koguryo. This life taught him, through the painful experience of losing all he had and the family he loved by the hands of one power hungry man, that social status and possessions do not mean much.

Though superficial memories in our consciousness get altered and distorted as time goes by, the memories and emotions in our subconscious seem to stay intact through long period of time. Especially, strong emotional contents of the memories retain their specific energy characters and information contained in them unchanged. Hypnosis enables us to reach those subconscious memories that are repressed and hidden from our superficial consciousness, to find solutions of current problems. If we developed efficient ways of utilizing patient's subconscious memories and potential abilities, we will be able to find solutions to many of the difficult symptoms. After leaving the life in Koguryo behind, we rested for a few minutes. When we set out to find another life of Won's past, he became a sheepherder in Scotland.

W: I am in a wide open field...There are sheep... It is Scotland...

K: What are you doing?

W: ...I am a sheepherder...

K: What clothes are you wearing?

W: ...I am wearing only one piece garment... It is made of leather and the top and bottom are connected...

K: What is your name?

W: ...McConell...

K: Is it your last name?

W: ...They just called me by that... I don't know if it is last or first name...

K: How old are you?

W: Thirty six

K: Do you have family?

W: ...I have a wife, a daughter and a son...I have another lover too...

K: Your wife's name?

W: She is called... 'Suzina'

K: What is the name of your lover?

W: ...Mica or Mita...

K: When is this?

W: ...In 1,200s... It is very difficult for folks like myself to live due to heavy taxes...Herding sheep is my work...The sheep belonged to the lord...I am very poor and it is hard to live without stealing...

K: Do you know what region of Scotland it is?

W: ...West side of Scotland...I think they are calling it 'Burmesett... (the pronunciation was not clear whether it is 'Bermesett' or 'Burmeseck')

K: Can you tell me the exact year? (I instructed him to concentrate after brief relaxation)

W: ...I see the figures... '1231'...

K: Can you tell me your full name?

W: ...No last name...I was just called McConell...

K: What are the names of your children?

W: My daughter is 'Tipi' and son 'Harris'...

K: Do you have many neighbors?

W: There are many people like us... I tend the lord's sheep and receive grain ...but it is not enough...

K: Is your family happy?

W: ...No... my wife is very jealous because of my lover...

K: How did you meet your wife?

W: We knew each other since we were very young...

K: Did you love your lover more than your wife?

W: No...I don't think so...It is just my wife is necessary in the household... and I needed the lover as a companion for me to relax...

K: Is your lover married too?

W: No...

K: Will you go to a time when your family is together?

W: ...I call my son 'Harry'...and I used to hit him a lot...I drink heavily too...

K: You don't love your family?

W: ...There wasn't much to call 'love'...I behave as I please... I am rough and reckless.

K: Let's move to an important scene in that life...

W: ...I am very good at stealing...I stole anything that was worth money, and later I stole anything for curiosities' sake and threw it away...

K: Did everyone steal?

W: ...Yes, whenever possible...and everyone tried hard not to be stolen...

K: Let's move to the next important scene...

W: (In a very small voice) ...I am now trying to rape my own daughter...

K: How old is she?

W: Sixteen... My sexual desire was too strong... I was looking for a new partner... then I took an interest in my daughter...

K: Is your daughter's name Tipi?

W: ...Yes...when she was young... but now she is called 'Jamie'.

K: Let's go forward in time...

W: (after a short pause)... I didn't feel too pleasant... But I didn't get punished at all because of that...

K: What were your feelings?

W: ...I regretted a little bit...but I didn't anguish over it...

K: What was your daughter's reaction?

W: She resisted at first but gave it up at the end...she is crying now...

K: How old are you now?

W: ...Over forty years old...

K: Let's move to the next important scene...

W: ...I think it is when I am dying... I am eating a poisonous plant...it is painful...The plant has nothing to do with my death... I don't know why I ate it... (after a brief pause)... Ahh!... (moaning as if in agony)...Someone stabbed me in the back with a spear...

K: Who stabbed you?

W: Someone with hatred of me...He is the husband of someone I had slept with...

K: Is it much painful?

W: ...There is no pain...I can see myself with eyes open; glaring...I am fifty three years old...

K: Can you tell me of your appearances?

W: ...Long hair...bold and mean face...

K: Relax a little and pass through the moment of your death... (after a short while) Where are you now?

W: I don't know... It is just a dark place...

K: Can't you see yourself?

W: No, I don't see anything...

K: What is the meaning of that life time?

W: ...About love... I realized at the moment of my death that I had committed enormous wrongdoing too often...a big change occurred...

K: What change is it?

W: ...I obtained a higher consciousness that I hadn't had while living... I am now able to see what I did wrong objectively...

K: Is someone teaching you?

W: No...The realization...came to me suddenly...Oh! ...Someone is talking to me now...

K: Listen to it, what does it say?

W: (in a low, very calm tone, completely different from Won's own voice)

Yes... It is... At times, the life given to us can become like this as well...Those events which visit us every moment of our life may lead to a realization or may not...Why do people realize their sinful deeds only after their death?... Please, have eyes… Have eyes in your present life that can correctly see what you should truly pursue in your life and what kind of life you need to live... Otherwise, you will only repeat endless remorse...Please, live with deep empathy... The eyes that can see correctly through life start from innocence...The reason why who help others get to possess clearer soul is not because the behavior which help others make it to become so...but it is that his or her soul is getting disciplined through such behavior...the soul gets purified so... A good natured life may not change many things in life, but such a life is useful means...When you help others... it does not mean that the help you provide will bring you certain reward...It is only that your soul gets to open its eyes and grow in the process of helping others... (in a loud and strong tone)...Who feels the most severe guilty conscience?... One that practice evil does not feel compunction... One that practices goodness does... However, even if you practice evil, it does not mean that the value of your soul diminishes due to your act... Please, open your eyes... Live every moment in emphatic passion...

The Voice ended here. When I woke Won up after having him rest awhile, he said with a confused expression on his face "It was the voice of a very kind woman this time. It was thick male voice last time, they are totally different..." He said that he did not remember every detail of the message spoken through him but he could recall the general content of the message.

Although most of the people who have experienced Past-Life Regression speak of the teachings and realization they felt in their past lives, this style of lengthy and analytical interpretation through the Voices of the Wise is quite a rare phenomenon. Teachings of most religion are love, compassion, overcoming of anguish through realization and return to Truth. But the teachings of the Voice seem a little different from those of religions because the Voices emphasized and described love and sacrifice as the universal virtue that is more than a religion. For reasons that both of us didn't understand, the Voices were revealing much to us with deep compassion.

CHAPTER 5

The Fourth meeting:

Africa, the World after Death and the Prophesy for the Future

Before we began the fourth regression after a week, I asked Won briefly about how he was doing in his personal life. "I think a significant change is happening in my life. I used to not be able to forgive other's errors, but such repulsion has disappeared...and when I try to see through to their souls, I feel so much peace inside... I actually feel compassion and sympathy toward them...What I felt about the life of McConell was that the soul which realized itself first is not necessarily the better one...I felt that each soul is equally precious...recently, I do not feel any more abhorrence I used to have against China...They are completely gone... I feel there will come some change in general direction of my life... Now, I feel I can caress my own soul... I would like to concentrate my efforts on what's really important."

The seventh life was in Africa. When I instructed him to go ahead after guiding him into deep hypnosis, we met a Masai warrior.

K: What do you see?

W: ...I am a Masai warrior...I am armed...

K: What kind of weapons do you have?

W: ...Shield and spear...

K: Where are you?

W: ...Africa...I see mountain Kilimanjaro...

K: What is your name?

W: ...Undihte

K: Undihte, is it your name?

W: Yes...

K: What do you look like?

W: ...I am a Masai warrior...

K: Please, describe your appearances.

W: ...Short hair...protruding cheekbone… and elaborate ornaments... I am about 180 centimeters tall...

K: Are there other warriors around you?

W: No...

K: What are you doing?

W: ...It is just an ordinary day...I am not doing anything special...I am touching up ornaments on my weapon and my body...

K: Do you have family?

W: Yes...I have parents, a young brother and other siblings... there are six of us...

K: What is the year?

W: It is in the 12th Century...

K: Are there many people living in your village?

W: About one hundred to one hundred fifty... My clan is medium to medium large in size... not very large one.

K: Is there a name for your village?

W: ...No specific name for the village... but our clan is called by a name that means 'Brave Masai'.

K: Let's proceed to another scene...

W: ...Because I was, a weak hearted as they say... an easily scared person... I was teased and ridiculed much by many... many singled me out...I would often be in a difficult spot when in hunting...because I was not doing well in hunting... That's what I was... There is an old man in our village...he was called the 'Wise One'.

K: Where is your family?

W: (After brief silence)... I don't see them...

K: Shall we go to the next important event?

W: (in small voice)... I killed a friend...

K: Why did you kill him?

W: He had always made a fool of me and abused me... so I quickly stabbed him with a spear... (the tone of his voice was rather indifferent but thrilled)... Village neighbors and elders told me to leave the clan...

K: How old are you?

W: About forty years old...

K: So, what did you then?

W: ...I wandered around empty fields...starved... shivering from cold air at night...

I often longed to see my children ...(after long silence)...I don't think I lived long from then on...

K: Did you die wandering in the open?

W: ...Yes...

K: What do you look like?

W: ...Crouched into a ball...a very gaunt man is lying on the ground... I am looking at him...

K: Are you already dead?

W: Yes...

K: Where are you now?

W: ...I am right next to my corpse looking at it...

K: What do you feel?

W: ...Not much, freed from my sinful deed... I feel no joy of freedom after death... rather, I feel oppressed... there are things I cannot escape from...

K: Is there much remorse about the things you could not do?

W: ...No, there isn't...

K: Where do you go from there?

W: ...I am now rowing a boat... crossing a river... I see two persons...

K: (confused momentarily) ...Are you in another life?

W: No... I am dead and crossing the river... Two persons in white dress are here to greet me...

K: Do you know them?

W: No...

K: What kind of river is it?

W: ...River of Death...of course...

K: Do Masais cross the river when they die?

W: ...Every one of us crosses it when dead...

K: Did the two persons bring the boat to greet you?

W: They are not persons...but Spiritual Guides... one of them tells me that I took much trouble and the other stares me with a reproaching look...

K: Did it take much time crossing the river?

W: ...No it didn't...

K: What are your surroundings like?

W: ...I can't see anything...

K: Can you see the water?

W: ...Even the water is black... K: What shape is the boat?

W: ...It is similar to a rowboat we ride...but it is only a boat in the realm of consciousness... the boat doesn't exist in reality...

K: Then, It is a symbolic boat?

W: Yes...

K: Where are you going now?

W: ...I am accompanying the two guides... I just entered a village... The goal is to learn anew...

K: Are there many people in the village?

W: The village is not for people... but for souls... those two who greeted me are the leaders here...

K: What do you learn in the village?

W: Our own deeds... We get to review our actions in life and reevaluate them... we view them again and contemplate... We frequently submerge in lengthy contemplation... No happiness nor sadness there... it is not a place to feel emotions...Without changes in emotion we look back and contemplate there... and plan and meditate on the life to come...

K: Do you see any familiar faces there?

W: ...There are no faces here...

K: Can't you identify others?

W: ...We can identify one another...but there is not much significance in doing it because we all look the same here...

K: Have you met anyone you knew in life?

W:... I sense a familiar person... Park...he is one of my junior at work... I seem very exhausted and... this is a place with little emotion...

K: Is it a place just for learning?

W: ...Yes...

K: What did you learn from Undhite's life?

W: ...Once again, I felt with bone-aching pain, how important a life is...

Have the determination to endure... not avoiding... (in a painful tone)... it is very difficult to continue...

K: Okay...Where do you go when the learning is finished?

W: ...We don't have much right to choose, and we must leave again whether we want it or not...

K: You must return to this world?

W: Yes...We don't know when, but we must return to earth whenever we should...that is a matter for the highest God to decide...

K: Did you suffer any punishment for killing a friend?

W: The punishment there... a mental anguish is the punishment there...

K: Are your own deeds the cause of anguish?

W: The wrongdoing I committed in life becomes a heavy yoke that feels so tormenting... feels like I am completely bound by it...Certain deeds feel much more painful and burdensome than others...This is the place where those evil deeds we commit in life torment us so that we cannot rest comfortably...

K: Is this a place of unending discomfort?

W: ..I don't feel any peace nor happiness there... I need to learn fast enough... that is most important there...

K: Very well... We will proceed to next scene...

W: Hmm... Someone is talking to me.

K: Listen to it...What does he say?

W: (in a solemn voice)...The pain you receive is suffered inside... in the realm of your soul... Even if you are maltreated by others, you should not hate, nor curse the others... because they are not the ways to solve the problem... instead; it becomes a yoke which binds you further... If someone tries to hurt you, let yourself be hurt... It will rather free your soul...If you see a soul who tries to trouble and strain you, do not attempt to fight it... Such a confrontation will make your next life more difficult... Instead of concentrating on what distresses you, focus your efforts on the proceedings to your perfection... There are many powers that restrain you from reaching the Truth...You cannot reach the Truth by troubling or entertaining yourself... Do not commit wrongdoings and such ways of life that can obstruct your soul's freedom...Expand your mind by having true freedom...and contain as many people as you can in it...Forgiveness is the true freedom. One who has the Truth can forgive, and one who can forgive will become free...Do not try to possess...All problems arise from possessions... When relieved from the obsession of possessing, you will be freed from the binds of hatred and evil... Give... the space left empty by giving will be filled with freedom...

Revel in true freedom...Do not try to get consolation or help from other people... they will get in the way of your growth...Look inside of you and do the things that will help your soul to stand by itself...No one can harm or harass you except yourself because you are already in the realm of God... The only one who can destroy you is yourself... thus, do not hate those who try to distress you, destroy you or steal what you possess... Distinguish reality from illusions and do not chase after illusions... The deeds of hatred toward you, the minds that harass you are all illusions... See through the constrained minds of those who hate you...and focus on the binds on their souls...they are reality... When you do not focus on the sins and see the souls behind it, your soul will expand without limits...your freedom will become boundless...Do remember this Truth... This is the end...

K: Has the Voice stopped?

W: Yes...

K: Has it gone?

W: ...It has not gone away ...I only heard it...

K: Can I ask the Voice?

W: Yes...

K: Where do the obstructing powers that hinder us from reaching the Truth come from?

W: (solemnly, the Voice resume the talk) ...The realms of Good and Evil spirits actually exist... The evil spirits manipulate and urge you to focus on the Illusions, not to focus on the Real. You think it justice when you scrutinize, curse, reprimand and judge those who hate you and rob you of your possessions and positions... But that is not justice... True Justice is the insight and the power that enable you to escape the temptation and insinuation of the evil spirits and make you see the essence of your own soul. When you possess such spiritual powers, you can overcome the influence of evil spirits... Do not be fooled by the evil spirits that tempt and anger you... Truly, in the realm of the spirits, there are darkness and light, goodness and evil, temptation and righteousness... Many assume that establishing a Justice is the most righteous, but it is not so... The justice you stand by, or the religious doctrines you believe in are actually proceedings toward a new form of possession... Do not possess... The road you can take to avoid temptation is not to possess... The Voice ends here...

K: Can we know the essence of ourselves?

W: The essence of yourself is life...Every life form has its value and nobility... Life does not bear itself, it is born. In other words, there is a being that created you...There is a being that created humankind, spirits and every living thing... He had made them all...We are his creation, but at the same time, we are a part of him... Thus, you cannot become God, but you can become a part of God... This is the essence of life... God has allotted his life to you... Your life and the life of a cricket are given from the God... The Voice ends here...

K: Where do the evil spirits come from?

W: ...The evil spirits exist on a fixed time limit... They are similar to the dirty plates before being cleansed in water...The evil spirits are the tools temporarily used to complete your spiritual perfection...They will exist and be active until every soul achieves its perfection...When the last soul reaches its perfection, the evil spirits will disappear without trace, as they arose from the void in the beginning ...Everyone is like a passenger in the train bound for Truth... Although the first carriage arrives at platform first, the last one will get there also...No matter how evil a person is, he is on the train...When the train reaches the Truth, the evil influences disappear naturally...Do not focus on the realm of Evil...Why focus on the things that will perish?...See the everlasting ones... When you observe the everlasting, the evil will fall away...

K: Do you mean that we can win over the evil by focusing on the everlasting?

W: (in a gently reproving tone) ...You cannot win, you can only proceed...

K: Is this the end of the Voice?

W: Yes.

K: Are you very tired?

W: ...I feel a bit shaky...

K: Why do you feel shaky?

W: The energy in me is depleted from communing with the Universal Voice. And it hasn't been restored yet...

K: Then, we will rest and relax awhile...

W: (After about one minute, with a slightly excited voice)... There are many people around me...

K: Who are they?

W: They are not people. They are spirits, very advanced spirits.

K: Are they surrounding you?

W: Yes, they are staring at me...

K: Do they speak to you?

W: ...Some are looking at me kindly... and some try to tell me something...I feel like they will answer me if I ask them questions...

K: Do you have any question to ask?

W: ...I don't know... (after a brief pause)...They are telling me something... about arrogance...They tell me not to be arrogant...The true value is in a paradox, they say...They say that I should focus on the life that results from paradox...When I empty...I will be filled...When I fill, I become more impoverished...It may seem that sharing will make me depleted...but more will come when I share... When you humble yourself... (in an enraptured voice) ...There is no one who can block the light which shines from you... You should sacrifice and lower yourself, how valuable and beautiful is such a life...but there are too many who live in illusions of self-satisfaction... and they lower themselves with hidden arrogance... They suddenly tell me that Cardinal Kim (a religious leader of Korea)... can die next year... or his physical health will deteriorate severely...There will be many changes in 1997...

K: Continue, please...

W: They say, more and more people will get interested in the spiritual world in coming years...Now is a time of adjustment... There will come many difficulties, but people will learn the emptiness of possession through them... and will see more of the spiritual side of their lives... but the evil and tempting forces will also be rampaging more than before... What many religious figures have veiled for their selfish greed will be unveiled gradually...Since they don't comprehend the core of the Truth and see only the surface of the Truth, their authority will diminish... They can never be the messengers of the Truth... Yet, because they still hold the hegemony, they will oppress the people of Truth and those who search the road to Truth... Hence, many good people will be called insane...Since others don't know them, they will believe the virtuous to be insane when authority tell them so... This doesn't mean all the believers of cults and strangeness are virtuous...Time will become chaotic that It will be very difficult to distinguish good from evil... However, there is one measure to tell them apart... Judge whether the virtuous things you pursue are for your own pleasure, or are they for the benefit of the many... Be attentive to the things you pursue... Are they for self-satisfaction, or for others? Are they for the Truth or for our intellectual satisfaction, physical comfort, or fulfillment of curiosity?... There will come the time when it becomes difficult to tell truth from evil due to too many chaotic forces... We may live in a materially more plentiful world... but the life will become more barren spiritually... Hence, those who have the Truth will often be cast out from the society... But it will be only temporarily...Those outcasts will become the new hope of the coming era... This new era doesn't mean the New Age Movement... It is a time period in preparation of the opening of the World of Truth... The Voice ends here...

K: Are you still with them?

W: Yes...

K: Can I ask what will become of Korea in the future?

W: ...It will become an ethical nation... Much of Christian influences will diminish and dwindle...This does not mean that the Christian teachings has its limits... it is to say that those who hold power and authority in Christian churches but do not comprehend true Christianity...will fall...The bubbles disappear and only the grain remains...Buddhism will go the same way... Firstly, new figures will arise in religions... Secondly, nature-friendly movements will become more active, protecting and tending to nature; this movement will gradually strengthen over time... Thirdly, there will be preparations for spiritual phenomena...Mass production will not be as great as it has been...though its momentum may carry on for a while... material affluence will not guarantee the flourishing of the society ...Instead, the coming days will be such that spiritual life, ethical life, spiritual pursuit will enrich our cultures and lives...Those with political power will not prevail, but those with different values will... The new sort of political power that everyone dreamed of, will make the society happy... Now is the time of chaos before it... Unless we undergo this era, the new one will not arrive for a long time... The Voice ends here...

K: Could you tell me something about the prophecy of Nostradamus that says the world will end in 1999?

W: ...The end will come, but the course is different. The timing is different too. I can talk only this much...

K: Do you hear any other talk?

W: They show much interest in my person...

K: Do you see any familiar face?

W: ...I feel like that I probably was one of them in the past... I feel very friendly toward them...

K: Could they have come to visit an old friend?

W: It could be that or... it might not be that...

K: Are they still around?

W: Yes... They don't want me to continue any more today...

K: We will end here today... relax and rest...

The fourth session was very remarkable. Won remembered his period and the purpose of the realm where he went after death. The place of solitude and regret, to which he had to go due to his wrongdoing while alive, might be the hell or limbo about which we have often heard of. While there, he met again Park, Won's co-worker who had lived with Won as a young Buddhist priestess in Won's first past-life he remembered. The Karmic relationship between them must be very strong. After spending his due time in the place where his soul reevaluates its former life and plans the next life, Won departed to seek a new life. This seems to support a theory of transmigration that says 'Each soul departs anew to find the parents and environment that suit the growth of each soul the most.' The theory also states 'If you are born into an impoverished and difficult environment, it is because your soul needs such problems in this life to grow.' It seems that the basic elements of the next life are decided in the greater frame of our spiritual growth, and the specifics and details are influenced by our Karma. We all know the pain that arises inside us when we try to fight against the life's difficulties and conflicts with hostility and resentment. The theory of transmigration and Karma teaches us that this suffocating pain is a necessary process for our soul's growth.

The Voices taught us how to understand the pain in life, and proceed in perfecting our souls. They also emphasized the reality of the evil forces that try to keep us from reaching perfection and how we should overcome them. They answered some of my questions and, quite unexpectedly, gave us various prophesy regarding the future of our world. They all seem to contain significant messages.

Though we heard the Voice in the last three sessions, this was the first time the Voice told so much. I became a little excited but questions also arose in me. Won, who conveyed the long message had a mystified expression on his face when awoken from hypnosis. Most patients in hypnotic past life regression therapy show increase in insight and understanding, they understand and see their life remembered in therapy more objectively than when in normal consciousness.

Many realize and talk about the meaning and the purpose of the life. But only very few heard the Voice of Wisdom and conversed with it.

Catherine, whom Dr. Brian Weiss met is a very rare case. However, Won, conveys us more various and deeper Voices than Catherine did. I calmed my excitement, thinking it a great fortune to have met someone like Won. Though I didn't quite understand what he meant when he said 'probably I was one of them', in later session Won told me that highly advanced spirits also can reincarnate on earth, and there are people among us who possess such souls. I thought Won may be one of those advanced souls reincarnated.

CHAPTER 6

The Fifth Meeting:

Eighth life and its teachings, and Prophesies

We were back to the Chosun Dynasty, Korea, in Won's eighth life

K: Where are you?

W: ...I can see Kumgang Mountain (Diamond Mountain in North Korea)...

K: Can you tell me your appearances?

W: I am a Buddhist monk...

K: How old are you?

W: Fifty-two... I wear monk's clothing and conical bamboo hat for monks...

K: What is your name?

W: ...Yujung or Hyujung

K: Are you a man or a woman?

W: ...I am a male monk...

K: What are you doing there?

W: I... was discharged from the temple...I am traveling all over the entire Eight Provinces of Korea...subsisting completely on donations from other people...

K: Why were you discharged?

W: ...They said I tried to befriend a woman...

K: When were you discharged?

W: ...When I was just over forty years...

K: What was the name of your temple?

W: It is called Donghaksa... in Kyeryong Mountain...

K: What year is it?

W: ...Early 19th Century...

K: Where is your home town?

W: ...Haman...South Kyungsang Province...I became a monk in Hein Temple when I was young... I was told to become a heroic monk like Samyung during the Japanese invasion in 16th Century...I stayed there for a long time...I also stayed at another temple called Bumuhsa... My duty at Donghaksa was to teach people... but that ended...

K: Were you discharged due to a scandal?

W: (in a tragic tone)... It was more of a misunderstanding than a scandal. I just didn't try to explain it to justify myself...

K: What misunderstanding is it?

W: It is a misunderstanding that I tried to befriend a woman... I did not do that... I only tried to lighten her distress...

K: Why was she distressed?

W: ...She could not bear a child...She asked for my help... She thought she might become to be able to bear a baby if I placed my hand on her belly... it was not because she loved me... She just thought somehow I possessed mystical power...

K: What was her family name?

W: Sung...originally from Hehju... She is a descendent of a noble family...

K: What is your Buddhist name?

W: ...It is Yujung

K: What was your feeling when discharged for that reason?

W: (in a grievous tone)... It was oppressing... painful...

K: Why didn't you explain yourself?

W: ...I didn't want to put her in an awkward position... I chose to close the matter by bearing all the responsibility myself...

K: How did you feel while traveling around...

W: ...I felt like I finally found Buddha himself...

K: How was the society like then?

W: ...Much of the traditional orders had crumbled away... Those with enough money bought noble positions illegally...the value of noblemen had dropped much... economy was not very bad...

K: A relatively stable period?

W: Yes...

K: What were you doing near the Kumgang Mountain?

W: ...It is the time to prepare for the departure...

K: Where are you going to go?

W: ...It is time to close my life...

K: Proceed, please.

W: I see myself sitting in a small temple...

K: How is your appearance?

W: ...I feel, I possess a clear soul... I am fifty two years old.

K: What year is it?

W: ...1842...

K: Are you ill?

W: I grew weaker physically, but I feel more that the time has come...

K: Let's proceed... What do you see?

W: I see myself... My face is peaceful, smiling...

K: Where are you?

W: I am still sitting in the small temple... I slipped out of my body...

K: Where are you going?

W: ...I see white color all around me... I am riding on the back of an ox. The ox is going somewhere...I am going slowly on the back of the ox... to where I am supposed to go...

K: Is the ox in the spiritual world?

W: Yes...

K: Where is your destination?

W: ...It is the place they call 'Nirvana'...

K: Is your mind at ease?

W: No... I feel uneasy...

K: Why?

W: ...People, left behind... things, left behind...

K: What have you learnt in that life?

W: ... I am not sure...

K: Is there anything especially remorseful in that life?

W: ...It was a stage to prepare...

K: What did you prepare?

W: ...Prepared to lead many people to spiritual peace... through my inner power...

K: Is that the purpose of that life?

W: (in a resolute voice)... You could say so...

K: Let's proceed...

W: ...I arrived at a gate...

K: What kind of gate is it?

W: ...It is similar to that of a traditional Korean house... but the gate is not a physical one... it is a gate within my mind...I hear sound of chanting sutra... I smell incense...

K: Are there people inside?

W: ...The number 42 appears in my mind...

K: What does that mean?

W: ...It indicates the level of spiritual advancement... I feel it represents the level of my enlightenment... but I am not sure...

K: What more do you see?

W: ...I see a vision of myself re-entering a woman's womb...

K: Are you coming back right away?

W: ...I don't know...

K: Let's proceed...

W: Ah... Someone is talking to me...

K: Listen to it.

W: ...Our lives are not run precisely... Don't try to clarify yourself and don't try to fix yourself in a frame... When you fix yourself in a form, you are being confined... (in a whispering voice)... To become a bowl to contain the souls of people, you should not be confined in a form...Even with good intention, do not be confined in any fixed frame... We must see our essential appearances... Do you feel stressed because something is harassing you? ...Is other people's judgment on your social status and relations hurting you? ...The people's evaluation of others, admiration and obsession, are the products of illusion... Illusion creates greed, and greed produces jealousy and obsession... Those will bring difficulty not only to you but also to many others... and consequently, you will become disconnected and estranged from the truth...Do not create a fixed form and reside in it... To be free from a fixed form, we must be able to console ourselves from our chagrin... The best training for not confining ourselves in a fixed form is to love the soul of the one who hurt us...and understand his point of view even in your painful situation...That is, indeed, a starting point... Why do many people live exhausting lives? ...It is because they are chasing illusions... At times, we should be able to pray for our accuser's soul... ...It will be a starting point for an immense change... This is the end...

K: Where does this Voice come from?

W: ...It seems like; someone is talking right next to me...

K: Is it an interpretation of the life we saw?

W: Yes...

K: Did you feel much chagrined in that life?

W: Yes...

K: Although you did not explain yourself, you must have suffered a lot...

W: ...I thought I managed to control myself well enough, but I must have suffered a lot inside... (after a brief pause, the Voice returned, in a deep voice)... Let us view this... In order to embrace other people's pain, we must suffer the pain first...We can understand other's experiences by experiencing various lives ourselves...Do not try to overcome, try to embrace... Do not try to explain, try to understand... Voice ends here...

K: Is the Voice still next to you?

W: ...I think so...

K: Relax and rest...

W: (after about 30 seconds)... I hear the Voices again... They are chanting a sutra... K: Are you still in front of the house?

W: No... I am in the middle of the Universe...

K: Do you hear anything else than the chanting sutra?

W: (the Voice speaks)... A greater being is contained within a smaller be-ing, and the greater being is a part of the smaller one...The Universe is only a dot...and these dots gather to become even greater Universe...There is no beginning as there is no end...Who is Buddha?...The one who has Buddha's mind is Buddha himself... Small Buddhas gather to become a greater Buddha... and the Buddha of the Universe is within each person... Thus, a small being contains a greater being, and a greater being embraces a small being... Each life is put together to become a part of the highest God of the Universe, and the God dwells in each and every life form... What is the beginning?, and what is the end?... By possessing, you start a beginning, and when you release, a new beginning starts... Strive to love souls, and try to see the God who dwells in them... Idolizing a person makes you most unhappy...When you idolize someone, you cannot see the God within you... and You cannot discover the God within that person... Instead, you only focus on the image, created from people's greed including yours... In the opposite manner, this also applies to a villain... When you concentrate on the sins of a villain, you will miss his soul and the voice of God within his heart... You will only see the image, created by his sins... What is right and wrong? ...If you don't see the God in everyone, there is nothing different when you see one as a good person, for he did something nice to me, and seeing another as a bad one for he did something bad to me... It is the same because you only see images created by results of one's action, whether good or bad...You must see the God dwelling within...You must be able to see the greater being embraced within a smaller being, and while seeing the greater being, you should not forget that it is contained in a smaller being. (in an emphatic tone)... Without realizing this, you are not able to love a soul... the Voice ends here...

K: Are you still in the Universe?

W: No, I came back to myself...I see piano keyboards...

K: Where are you now?

W: This is a new metaphor... An explanation of the theory of Trinity is being revealed to me... The Voice is telling me that Trinity and the relations among people in a society have same principles... Each key looks the same on a keyboard, but each produces a different sound. From the lowest note to the highest, the musical pitches sound different. but we call all the notes and pitches the 'Piano sound'.

Yet, when the notes are played carelessly, without following fundamental rules of music, we don't refer the sound as 'performance', nor do we call it 'real piano music'...However, when the sounds make certain harmony, it becomes a piece of 'piano music'. Though each key and string may have its own note and good physical quality, the 'piano music' emerges only when the sounds make good harmony. In musical harmony, a totally new set of values resonate. Music is a new set of values beyond the sound of each and every key and string; it is out of the realm of the key and string's physical quality, though it may still be confined to the physical realm... This is a metaphor of our need to love our souls to become one with others and make harmony with them, and this is also an explanation on Trinity... A piano cannot produce music by itself. It needs a performer, note, key and string. Only when they work together, a sound is made... To make the 'Do' sound, the performer must knock the 'Do' key, and it must strike the corresponding string at the same time...In order to produce one effect, three different parts must cooperate...Although each part has a different function, the sound of 'Do' cannot be made without their conjoined action... This is a short metaphor of Trinity... They are showing this to me in pictures as well...

K: Are there many of them around you?

W: Five or six of them are surrounding me again...

K: Are they still talking to you?

W: They are smiling at me. They make me feel at ease... And I feel they are kindly urging me to grow more in spiritual manner...

K: Are they talking about something to you?

W: ...They tell me not to worry about my family...They are telling me to praise the God... to worship God... I feel very happy and at ease...

K: Do they tell you anything else?

W: No... I would like to rest a little...

K: Then, relax and rest...

W: (after a short rest)...They are showing me a herd of sheep, and I hear them telling me to forgive the life of McConell...

K: Those sheep, from the life of McConell?

W: Yes...

K: Have you not forgiven his life?

W: ...I can't easily forgive my mistakes and faults...They tell me to let go of this part of my personality...and they are asking me what I have learned from my past lives...They tell me that it has been only one soul, my own, that lived those different lives, and they urge me to view others in the same way...I have been thinking about what I have learned in the past lives...now, I can say I have learned 'respect and love toward life'.

K: Now, do you feel all the different characters in the past lives are your own?

W: Yes...

K: Are the Voices still around?

W: ...I feel like, they care about me very much... It seems that they want to tell me about many things... but they don't do so, because they are afraid I am not able to take too much at one time...

K: Do you have anything to ask them?

W: ...Well... I'm afraid; I may become more arrogant because of their talks and love toward me... (after a brief pause)...You can ask questions...

K: Are they next to you?

W: Yes...

K: Ask them about your own future.

W: (as if talking to himself)...What shall become of my future? ...They say fifty percent of my life's sketch is already drawn...the rest, I must fill in ... They are talking about my choice...whether I desire a comfortable life, or a rather difficult one that can help others... though I am afraid, I would like to live the latter one...

K: Are they asking you this because they respect your own decision?

W: ...Yes... but I already know that they want me to live the latter one... They are telling me this... I'll be misunderstood by many, and be praised by many as well. They show me a picture of a famous Reverend and tell me that I'll live a life similar to his...they tell me about who can become a person to embrace many souls...

K: Is the Reverend doing well in his work?

W: No.

K: What is he doing wrong?

W: He is too humanistic... Of course, he has warm and innocent qualities in him, but he regards his own thoughts as those of the God's... This is his fault... It is deplorable that he comes up short in his depth of loving other's soul, although he tries very earnestly in this... Compared to others, you can say his soul is more advanced, but he is entangled in many relations that resulted from the images of illusion... It will become more difficult for him unless he escapes from those illusions...

K: What is the situation of Korean Catholic churches?

W: ...The Catholic Church is...like a chestnut partly eaten by a worm, some parts are still healthy, but other parts need to be cut out... Korean Catholic church is relatively clean but some others in the world are dangerous... They are even involved in the narcotics business... They protect those who handle drugs...Although they know it is not a good thing to do...their positions help them to justify their actions... most people don't know they are really evil characters...

K: Do the Catholic authorities know about this but turn blind eyes to it? What is the reason of this?

W: ...Because they need to operate the organization...

K: Do you mean Catholic Church is the organization?

W: Yes...

K: Is it because they need money?

W: ...Money and luxurious life... well... It seems they are attached more to their position, than luxurious life... Election of the Pope is not by spiritual authority of the individual, but by connection... The key to electing a pope is contained in the word 'connection'.

K: You mean it is human relationships that decide who will become the Pope?

W: Correct... It will be unlikely for the Papal lineage to continue to have many more Popes... Even if it does, the situation may possibly repeat that of Avignon...

(I thought he was referring to the incident of 'Avignon Captivity'. The Avignon imprisonment was the period in which the Roman Papal Court moved to Avignon in southern France from 1309 to 1377. During this period, the power of the Roman Catholic Church declined because the Pope was under the influence of the King of France. As Urbanus VI was elected the Pope in Rome in 1378, the French king appointed Clemens VII as the Pope and tried to secure the Papal Court in Avignon. Hence, two Popes existed simultaneously for a brief period of time.)

W: ...Currently, the position of the Pope in the Vatican is being challenged by a covert force...and there is another power that operates in the city of Vatican... This power works separately from that of the Pope, and it has become very dangerous... They (the other power) have long been connected to communists... though they themselves are not communists, to maintain their church organization; they have been connected to communists for a long time... There are many churchmen in lower offices who believed in the ideal of protecting Catholic Church in eastern European regions under communist rule. But, as you climb to the top, you find the leaders oppressed by the pressure of maintaining the organization...In the future, all religious organizations will become like this... So, it is not a commendable idea to become a religious leader... Instead, you should focus on the souls of people without being seen... The New Age people are also dangerous... They tend to become consumed by their ideology... Although their beginning was pure, they have gradually become drunk with their ideology... There will be many who expect with eagerness for a new and better religion to emerge... but the people with new ideas on religion will be rejected and persecuted because of their unfamiliarity, even though their ideas contain Truths...The time will be confusing like you look through a kaleidoscope... There will be those who are familiar and good, those who are familiar but bad, who are unfamiliar but good, and who are unfamiliar and bad... If you are asked to pick one from these four sets of people, you should pick those 'unfamiliar but good.'... There will come a movement to unify major religions in the world...They will try to negotiate in their authority, influence and purpose. They will try to create a federation of religions... but the biggest problem of this movement is that such a unity does not begin from the love of Soul and the passion for Truth. Instead, this solidarity starts from the anxiety of each religion to protect its invested interests, and keep the hegemony in its own territories... so, they will conspire with people of immense capitalistic influence... Ah... there are already huge flows of funds among hidden powers... people with religious authority, who are obsessed only in the images of illusion, will try to place themselves and their organization within this flow of funds in this emerging time of capital domination... Therefore, newly emerging oppressors and their organization will be justified and secure their positions with the help of religions... Such a pattern will become common, and will be referred to as 'Cosmopolitanism.' ...This, however, is only a new name for the new ruling class, and it may take its course in a less desirable manner than what capitalism did in the past... There is a danger of such movement's expansion if we do not cherish respect for Life and the pursuit of Truth in our hearts... But we can prevent such movements from emerging, if we reject it... Capitalism will crash soon and a new system will appear, and this will become a turning point that will decide the future of human kind...

K: What will be the future of North Korea?

W: North Korea will not perish easily... They will change gradually... They will unite with South Korea in a form similar to that of a federation... It will be done by people of Korean peninsula in rapid political shifts... In the future, Korea will ally with three northeastern states of China to make a kind of united system... Independence of Tibet is not in sight yet, but the north-eastern Asia, including Manchuria and its neighboring region will form an economic coalition within the next 100 years... The meaning of national boundaries will become obsolete... Instead, alliances based on Information and Capital will emerge... In North Korea, communists will gradually lose power as reformists arise, and they will try to establish relationship with the United States or Japan to seek their practical benefits... A new South Korean leader who can deal with the new political power of North Korea will appear in time...

K: What will be the future of Japan?

W: Although Japan will keep a position among leading nations of the world... but the years around 2050 will be their turning point... They are already on the downhill course...

K: What is the cause of its decline?

W: They have no ability to embrace others...

K: Is the land of Japan secure?

W: ...It will depend on the people who live on that land... The way how they live and the way how they think will decide it... The clear evidences of the real possibility... of the sinking of Japan will appear... They must convert soon...

K: Are you tired?

W: Yes...

K: Let's rest...

Many teachings and prophecies were given in this session, like the fourth one. The Voice told Won how to accept the chagrin, how to distinguish images from illusion and reality. Explanations about the great beings contained in small beings, small beings in greater beings, harmony and Trinity were given. The current problems of religions, possible future movements of religion and their problems, New Age movement, Future of North Korea, North-East Asia, and Japan were told by the Voices. When delivering these messages, Won's voice tone changed into very solemn and authoritative manner and regardless of the length of the sentence, there were no perceptible delays or discrepancies.

The vision of riding an ox to Nirvana, the image of a traditional Korean house, and the sound of chanting sutra confirm, once again, the theory that the after-death experiences reflect the person's cultural background in the life. Some people would think the messages are a little too Christian, but I think it is because Won is currently a Christian, and I also am familiar with Christian teachings. The Voices were giving us messages full of clearly universal Truth and values of beyond-religious quality in various but consistent explanations. I do not know where these messages come from. However, if these messages contain virtuous teachings, the Voices that deliver such message must be virtuous. And I believe the prophecies of our future are being delivered to benefit us as well.

How many in the world are fortunate enough, as it is with Won and me, to meet beings that tell about future and give answers to many difficult subjects of life with apparent good intention? Though we should have been joyous and excited at our unsought for fortune, we were silent facing each other after the fifth session. We probably thought the same thing in silence. 'Why are they telling these things to us?' I felt a little excited and anxious at the same time. I became a little afraid of the things the Voices might tell us in the coming sessions, because the contents of the message were getting more serious and surprising. But, on the other hand, as I saw a chance to experiment with the situation, I thought about compiling a list of things I always sought the answers for without success. All of us probably want to ask questions concerning ourselves when we meet beings who seem to have all the answers. I was not an exception. But I was more curious about why such messages were being given to me than asking for answers to my personal questions. I felt as if the situation was like some parcel very important was delivered to me due to a mix-up at the post office. I felt like

I was not the proper recipient because I believed such heavenly revelations and prophecy were for someone with innocence and purity of soul. At least, I knew I was not such a figure.

Though I wanted to ask some personal questions to the Voices, I decided against it because I thought my questions could distract and interrupt what they intend to deliver to us. So, I made up my mind to follow the course of the future sessions silently. However, to my surprise, the Voice knew my suppressed curiosity already and answered my unasked questions in the next session. It was an explanation of myself and the relationship between Won and me.

CHAPTER 7

The Sixth meeting:

My Past-life Relationship with Won, and more Teachings and Prophecies.

K: What do you see?

W: I see a flower garden...

K: Where are you now?

W: It shows the state of my mind...

K: What is the condition of your mind?

W: ...I hear the words...'My dear, beloved one... I love thee.'...

K: Who is speaking?

W: (in a powerful and solemn tone)... The Absolute one speaks...

K: Do you hear his voice?

W: Yes...he is a higher being than the Voices...

K: Do you see yourself?

W: Yes...I do. I wear a white garment; it indicates the state of my spirituality...

the material of it is almost transparent, and cannot be obtained on earth... I'm being praised, because my capacity to love souls is being expanded...I hear the words... 'The pain in you will be eliminated...' And he tells me to love you... He says you are my guide in this journey... I hear him telling much about you... He says you are a man of much inner struggle... He tells me you have almost passed the time of discord...and you have restraint of peace within you...although you have had many frustrations...but you are, nevertheless, a person who seeks goodness...Although the pain and scars are not removed completely yet, you are putting out the things you thought were unfortunate in your heart, one by one...and you pursue what's truly valuable... They urge me to work with you... In the previous lives...We were brothers once...we were very close...you were the elder... and I was the younger one... You died at thirteen years of age, and I died at fourteen... We were twins... We were so close... almost like one...

K: Where did we live?

W: Egypt...

K: When was this?

W: ...Around the third century...

K: Can you tell me of their names?

W: ...Depantor ...Lepaneo... We were children of a noble family... A horrible epidemic swept the area, carried by a sandstorm... The bad elements in the sandstorm, germs, contaminated water... thus, you died first...and I withered to follow you... (in a very painful tone)... I cannot possibly describe our parent's agony and anguish... Our father was a high priest... He worshipped Osiris... I see, before my eyes, many happy moments of that life...

K: What was the parent's name?

W: Mellokandor was father's name... mother was Tasia...

K: Could a high priest at the time have a family?

W: ...He was not supposed to...but he did... There were two types of high priests. One could marry, and the other could not... Our father was a high priest who could not marry... He loved his family very much... and he was a man of kind heart... despite his mental torments... he hid us well... You were a man of many wandering... You can soothe the wounds of many, because you have suffered many wounds yourself... You received wounds often while growing up... but the origin of your wound is long way before this life time... You have been accused at numerous times, lived a life of an imbecile...and especially, starved to death once and lived a mad life... However, all these painful lives occurred to you because you were an extremely good-natured person... Ah... I see a farmer... The image tells us to till the soil of our mind... Saying 'I have suffered so much, this must be enough.' Cannot be accepted... No matter how much the farmer tills the soil, small stones turn up endlessly... because of these small stones, plants can't root themselves in the soil and the farmer's toil becomes useless... You and I shared a life another time as well... It was in the 13th Century... I was a woman, and you were a man...

K: Where did we live?

W: France...Avignon...You were a very prominent Father at the time and I was only an ordinary nun... You even became a bishop, but I was excommunicated... We were never been formally husband and wife, but we had been so...Afterwards, I lived a severely solitary and lonely life...and you lived in emptiness shrouded in the splendor of your career... This led us to meet again... You are now learning how vain a worldly title and fame is...I see a turtle... (in a very deep and thick tone)... Life is like this...The steps of a turtle... A turtle strives and labors in each step. It's progress is really feeble... This is life... Would we reach the goal of our existence soon only because we made a step of progress in spiritual growth, or achieved something in our soul? ...It is not so... Even if our eyes are fixed on the goal in distance, our steps are painfully slow...And there are jags of rock and thorns of cactus on our path... Do you know what Elephant-turtle is? ...the long and drooping neck of an elephant-turtle... The elephant-turtle looks forward... However, before it reaches its goal, predators can eat it up or other animals eat all its foods... That is life... There are many things you cannot approach, even though you know about them... But you must realize, these unapproachable things support your current existence...You exist because you are imperfect... In other words, you don't need to be born if you were already perfect... You don't need to live in this limited existence... The precious soul in each of us, listen to the cry of the soul... The soul may be staring at the goal line, but our bothersome flesh hinders the advance of the soul... But do not grumble...do not lament about this limitation because that is what makes you stronger... What gives longevity to a turtle is its body that slows its walk... The progress of your soul is possible only because you are contained in your limiting body and life span...Hence, do not be afraid of your repeating lives' agony, nor lament over it... Without experiencing it, you cannot progress... I see a piece of pastry... a pastry crumbles into minute nutrients and be absorbed into your body, your soul must crumble from its original form to be absorbed into the body of many... At times, into a sweet appetite, and at times into a bitter mouth, your soul must crumble into fine nutrients to blend with other food to disintegrate in one's mouth, leaving no trace of its own taste... People call the final product of food, 'shit', and scorn its unpleasantness... They seldom appreciate the energy they received from consuming food... Suppose you sacrifice your soul to help and rejuvenate others... Will the recipients of your sacrifice thank you for what you did for them? ...Not at all... They may feel touched by what you did... but they will try to stay away from you because they think they will lose much when they accept and follow your sacrifice... Hence, those who sacrifice themselves to help others' souls will be despised and maltreated. Yet, how can food give energy without becoming 'shit?' ...When we truly give help to others is when we accept to make ourselves as low as 'shit.' ...What moves them and their bodies? ...The energy within you... Who consumes you is able to move because of your energy... But, of course, they would think they are moving by themselves... Teaching is, when the teacher becomes feces, convincing the students that they can do by themselves what they learnt... This is true 'guiding'... Yet, there is new life force in the feces... This is the end of the message... K: Where are you now?

W: ...I am in my consciousness...

K: Is there anyone around you?

W: ...I don't see any, (after a brief pause)...You must set up a base camp... Establish the base camp of your life... One who reaches the summit may become overjoyed by his own feat... but he could not have done it without the base camp...Who is more important person? The one who climbed to the top or the one who remained at the base camp? ...They both are important...The Voice ends here...

K: Is this all?

W: No... I need to rest awhile...

K: Then, relax and rest...

W: (suddenly, after resting about 20 seconds)... North and South Korea will be reunited after much twists and turns... I see many faces overlapped on the map of Korea... After the reunification, containing the tremendous amount of energy would not be easy... Siberia will come under the economic influence of Korea, but this will be different from other colonies managed by capitalistic nations... Spiritual influence of Korea will spread far and wide... Korea ought to become the nation which serves the rest of the world...In order to serve others, Korea has first given itself many wounds and scars... As one who never suffered pain cannot console other's pain, law and order cannot be established without first experiencing chaos... A great spiritual leader will emerge from this country...This does not mean no spiritual leaders will appear from other nations... China, India, France and Africa...from many countries, new leaders will arise... They are all born and alive already... but, their time of leadership will be thirty to forty years in the future... Look forward to this... The start of new theory may come from Korea... it does not belong to Korea... It belongs to the World... Do not take this in a foolish nationalistic point of view. No matter where it starts from, or who serves whom, the whole humanity must enjoy this together... The name of the Christ will shine even more... The Gospel of Jesus will overcome the religious prejudices, and will be sincerely accepted... All Truth will unite to become one, and all the teachings that assumed different shapes and forms for various people will become one as it used to be... This is the end of the Voice...

K: Is delivering the message more draining than watching images portrayed before your eyes?

W: No, it isn't... I am like a computer with the power cord connected... There may appear nothing on the screen, but a lot of processes are going on inside... My condition is especially good today... So many messages are pouring into me that I can hardly rest... (after being silent for about 30 seconds) ...I see my heart... There is yellowish fat on the walls of my heart... To eliminate this, I have to change the frequency of the vibration of my body... Nowadays, doctors are using chemicals to dissolve this away... but there will be new methods of treatment available... The differences in the frequency of atomic vibration in cholesterol and my cells will create friction to prevent cholesterol from sticking to the wall of blood vessels... Therefore, the cholesterol will be washed away... Yet, in order to make this happen, people will have to live more spiritual lives... When we become able to create higher spiritual vibration, all the harmful virus and bacteria will be washed off as well... Hence, a noble soul will create as noble a body... This kind of medicine will be possible after the year 2050... One profession that will disappear in that future, unfortunately, is psychiatrist. Many spiritual leaders will improve and refine the skills and arts already known to men...

Medicine at this time will not be bound to chemicals as Western medicine is now, nor will it depend on the 'force' as Eastern medicine does. Instead, it will take care of our souls as well as bodies at the same time... Disease will be washed away by the vibration of our souls... Hence, people will overcome the limits of their physical body, and their life span will increase accordingly... The mind will become the center of attention... The unknown realm of mind and soul will shed its shroud to reveal their mysteries to us... Logical positivism has already reached its end... Empirical science has reached a conclusion which is similar to agnosticism... In other words, logic of empiricism is not a reliable tool in unveiling mystery. There will be movements to discard empiricism... Why discard it? ...Because it does not have an accurate measuring standard... What is an accurate measuring tool? ...It is your soul and mind... When you have found a precise measure, you no longer need to use imprecise one... This is the end...

K: Rest and relax, if you want to... If you hear or see anything, you can proceed to tell me...

W: I see cows... There are many innocent souls gathered in Africa...The energy of their souls will be proven very valuable... Their child-like, innocent souls will work as energy to change the world... It is a miserable land now; we must protect it from being polluted further... The pollution by materialism there is growing day by day... but the innocent souls there must not be contaminated... And the souls of those who have lived hidden in the unknown Central Asia and Himalaya region will change the world with their vibration and frequency... Who are the people that live against the flow of the Universe, and who are the ones that go along with that flow? ...Who live according to the will of heaven is the person with vibration that is in tune with the Universe... Why do people cry out that humankind will perish? ...Because people detach their frequency from that of the Universe as the end draws near... People must match their frequency to that of the Universe, but as they don't know the frequency of the Universe, they are unable to do so... This mismatch will produce destructive force that will demolish the material-based civilization... But, those who have matched their frequency to that of the Universe will amplify the vibration of the Universe in the new spiritual civilization that comes afterward... This amplification of the vibration of the Universe will move many people in a form of moralistic influence, and those who do the amplification will have authority to become leaders... We may stop here today...

K: Are you tired?

W: No, I am not... But I hear them telling me to stop...

K: Alright... let's rest a while...

W: (after a short rest)... I see the past life when we were together... It's Egypt... Two children are playing around. They play with mud, and imitate sword fight with sticks... I see our mother coming over and patting us...

K: What do they look like?

W: ...They are adorable...

K: How old are they?

W: ...Six years old... dark complexion... You and I are now rising in the shape of angels... Ah... many images blend all at once...

K: Is the energy too strong?

W: ...Yes, I can't take it...

K: Erase all images from your mind and rest...

W: (after a short rest)... Images and Voices are being tangled... I feel my energy depleted... I'd better stop here today...

After he fully awoke from hypnosis, he told me 'I was hovering in the middle of the Universe and saw a magnificent view of it. I can't exactly describe the experience in words but I felt like I was in an I-MAX movie screen.' For the past five sessions, I led him through the process but he led me completely this time. I had no other choice than listening to his amazing stories. While doing past-life regression sessions with my patients, I also became a little curious of my past-lives. But I was always tired at the end of my workdays and I couldn't find time to do the regression on myself even on weekends because I was always busy. However, during the sixth session with Won, the Voice told me two specific stories of my past lives and other few hints. Since I never talked about my suppressed curiosity, the Voice must have read my mind to talk about my past-lives. The Voice might also have wanted to give me some assurances to my doubts in these regressions and messages. Another patient of mine once told me that she saw me in her past-life of several hundred years ago. Now I have heard about three different past lives of mine. Considering all the circumstances, I believe those stories are trustworthy because the people who told them to me were earnest and upright people and had no reason to fabricate such stories.

When I ask my patients how they can recognize people from their past lives who are also in the present life, they always answer, 'I just know.' It seems we have the innate ability to recognize the same soul in our sub-conscious level of mind. Patients refer to the stranger they didn't meet in past lives as 'I feel I don't know him at all.' Since my childhood, I have had my share of spiritual wandering, self-righteous and too independent way of thinking. This trait manifested itself as a never ceasing quest for the ultimate Truth, complete rejection of immoral authority, unyielding defiance against corrupt power, and co-existence of extreme self-control and self-indulgence. Though I have been lazy, self justifying and impulsive to do as I please in many things, the real core of my life have been extensive reading and thinking. Fundamentally, cold reasoning and empirical way of thinking suit me well and my personal conclusion on transmigration and the existence of souls was a completely logical product of contemplation after reviewing many evidences on the subject. Recently increasing reports of individual accounts of reincarnation that were supported by evidences also influenced my conclusion. As the things the Voice spoke about my past in this life were all correct, I think what it said about my past lives probably be correct as well. What the Voice told me, in a way, strengthened my faith in myself. If the teaching of Buddha, 'When your clothes merely graze that of a passing-by stranger, three past lives deep Karma is between you and the stranger.' were true, my patient Won, who came to me voluntarily to explore his past lives could have been my brother or lover in some of my past lives. What the Voice told us in this session covered many subjects - the agony of life and its reason, the futures of civilization, religion and medicine, the innocent souls in Africa and Central Asia, the limit of logical empiricism. I don't have anything to add to this message because the Voice was very specific about what it had to say. I leave the freedom to judge the contents to the readers.

CHAPTER 8

The Seventh meeting:

The Third Room, The meaning of this encounter, my problems, Spirit possession and Prophecy

The seventh session started in a strange atmosphere. For whatever reason, I felt vaguely uneasy from the beginning, and as if my inner insecurity influenced Won, I had to lead him longer than usual as he could not relax enough to go into deep hypnosis.

K: Do you see or feel anything?

W: I don't see anything... I hear someone telling you, 'Do not expect too much from this man.'

K: Who says that?

W: ...The one who protects me... It is the one who is always with me...

K: Is it a spiritual being that protects you?

W: Yes... It says 'This man must be protected more, needs to be hidden and protected.' ...and it suggests you regulate my breathing a little more...

K: How does it want me to do that?

W: …It suggests you lead me more softly…It asks you to lead me out the door once more…reverse the process of walking down the stairs…then proceed again in a more comfortable state… I feel I will see much today…but I am restrained…My heart beats very rapidly…

K: Erase all the images from your mind… and rest… go deeper into relaxation… We will rest until you feel comfortable to proceed…

For those readers who are not familiar with guiding techniques in hypnosis, I should briefly describe the process. Once the patient has been inducted into hypnosis, there are many ways to lead him into his past life memories. Although the choice of the method depends largely on the preference of each therapist or patient, I led Won down an imaginary staircase and had him open the door at the bottom - This door led him into his past life. So far, this method had always worked well with Won. But, in our seventh session, he asked me to reverse the usual process of climbing down the staircase and proceed once again from the top of the staircase. So, after relaxing a little more, I instructed him to exit through the door and climb the staircase.

W: …I can't climb up the stairs… Tell me to enter the 'Third Room'

K: (Though I was a little surprised and puzzled at this request, I followed his lead.) …Now, you can enter the Third Room…

W: …I just entered the room

K: What do you see?

W: (in a stable and calm voice) …This is the warehouse of Knowledge and Wisdom… K: Are you alone there?

W: …I am alone for now… but many have been here before…

K: Who have been there?

W: Those we call sages and prophets... have been here... This place is what you may call the 'Akashic Record'...

K: Is it the warehouse of Akashic Record?

W: ...Correct...

K: Why did you go in there?

W: ...To teach many things to many people...

K: Is this the protective spirit who's answering me?

W: (strongly) ...Yes...

K: What can we learn?

W: Through this encounter... you and this person will learn anew what is truly important in life...And you will know what to prepare for the time to come... Moreover you will be healed of your inner problems and conflicts through this person...

K: Are we supposed to contribute to the improvement of humankind through these meetings?

W: There is one condition if you wish to do so... You are not to privatize or use what you learn from your curiosity for your own fame or interest... You are to participate only with your child-like character that's inside of you...Yes... I know you have sincere interest in the souls of many, but you also have many wounds to be healed. Even if your theories are confirmed to be correct through what happens in these meetings, you should not be overjoyed or satisfied... Everything you learn from this process must be used to dissolve yourselves... It must be used to satisfy many...and in feeding many people, the universal Truth... This person really needs to be protected... The time is not his yet, but it will be so in ten or twenty years... be supportive of him, then... regard him like your younger brother, a friend or your student... You will have good relationship.. .Ah...I can see your mind... The entangled yarn and clear spring water...You still have problems to solve...You should become more honest...but I know you have endeavored much...Let us explore the Truth together... Ask questions if you have any...

K: Can you tell me about my brother?

W: ...Regarding him... there is resentment... and deep grief as well... Before my eyes, a vision of an immensely wide and open place is being formed... Now I am buried in the middle of the great field... and become an unnoticeable small dot... I don't hear any more words about your younger brother...

K: Is it better not to ask about my personal matters?

W: No... The Voice says the main problem is within me... Firstly, lack of confidence in me... Secondly, questions on personal matters may strengthen my conviction on the existence of spiritual world... but, it may lead to a wrong direction...

K: May I know the situations surrounding his death?

W: ...Such a wrongful death... Do you think your brother died of an accident?

K: No.

W: You're right.

K: Was he killed by someone?

W: It was such a rancorous death... Your brother seems to be a person who had been wrapped in anguish for a long time... Nonetheless, you should not harbor spite against those whom you think have killed your younger brother... Although your parents and your family have suffered a tremendous amount of anguish due to the incident... you must let go the spite...

K: What are the things I can do for him?

W: ...One who can untie a loop can untie ten and more... If there are people close to you who have hurt or complicated your life, forgive them first... place yourself in their positions, and see the matter with their eyes... If you do that, you will be able to forgive them... You are innately aggressive, but you get hurt easily... You know those opposite traits in you, are still causing pain... Is it not time for you to be changed through our messages? ...Remember the days when you caused pain to others, and suffered yourself in those relations... Truly, what caused you to make others painful were only trivial things... Yes... Depending on our point of view, a big problem can become small, and a very small thing can become a noose that immobilizes you... (in a loud and strong tone, rapidly)... You have to free yourself from the unexplainable anger and spite. The origin of those was your past-lives... You pacify the minds of many people, but you seem to become more and more skeptical in doing so...You need to unburden yourself of those empty feelings and inner anguish... You also need to be healed by these meetings... and you need to check the degree of change which will take place in you... Consoling other people without resolving your own grudge is likely to create only a shallow self-content... Suggesting others to drop their daggers without dropping yours first is only hypocrisy, falsehood and deception... The Voice ends here...

K: Are you still in that room?

W: I think so...

K: Am I allowed to ask any question?

W: ...I don't hear any answer, but I feel you can try...

K: Can 'Spirit Possession' actually make people ill?

W: (immediately)...Yes.

K: Are such illnesses common?

W: Yes... very common...

K: What is the remedy?

W: ...The most important reason of such 'Spiritual or Demonic possession' is that people do not forgive themselves and get extremely obsessed with things... Spiritual Possession occurs more frequently, when the victim's obsession and love-hate feelings attract the matching destructive energy from the Universe... than evil spirits torment the victim...

K: Do you mean when the victims free themselves from obsession, the so called evil spirits will scatter away?

W: Yes... It is not the victim expels the evil. When the good energy of the Universe, you may call it 'holy spirit', enters the body, the polluted energy has no choice but to exit...

K: Are all Spirit Possession a product of victim's mind?

W: Not necessarily so... Although most of the cases are made so... Powerful spirit can possess people, but such cases are extremely rare...

K: How do we solve such cases?

W: For now... you must wait...

K: Are these meetings meaningful for the benefit of other people, for preparing the future?

W: Yes... But this person must be protected... He must be protected now to work for a greater work in the future... He will be helpful in many ways to you... And both of you will be able to work together well by sharing the innocent minds of yours...

K: What will become of Israel in the future?

W: ...Blood... It can be called that... Israel... the images are becoming gradually blurred... Israel will have to pay for what wrong they have done... They shed too much blood... They unnecessarily shed too much blood because they do not want to compromise...They committed many crimes... They will have to pay for what they have done... Now, I feel I like to leave the Third Room...

K: Do they ask you to leave?

W: No...

K: Why do you want to leave?

W: I am afraid to stay.....

K: Are the images too burdensome?

W: It is not that...

K: Has time come to leave the Room?

W: ...No, It is because I have fear that I might undermine the authority of the Voice...

K: Are the Voices able to return to Earth?

W: ...There are some among Voices who work on earth at present... but they are not separate beings... They are of one complete being and they have simultaneity... They can exist in each other's mind... And they can exist as a separate physical being... What they refer to as the 'Holy Spirit' in Christianity, or the 'Merciful Heart of the Buddha' in Buddhism is in fact the Voice of Wisdom, or the work of advanced spirits...

K: What do I need to do to untangle the yarn and solve the conflicts in my mind?

W: ...You are doing quite well even now... You need to be freed from the memory of your childhood...

K: Does my aggressive tendency originate from my past lives?

W: ...It seems so... You were raised in a very noble way...But you once suffered a severe damage to your pride... (in a regrettable tone)... The hardened heaviness in your mind... I must say, came from that... You can be called a very fine person... but the frustrations you had while growing up... and a remaining fear about that memory is still in you... It is from your past life...

K: What can I do to help this person (Won)?

W: ...You need to see each other regularly... You may become a shelter for him to rest... As a counselor... or a friend to share spirituality ...It would be good to sustain such relationship with him...

K: Can I ask more questions?

W: If you were to ask...I might hesitate to answer... Confusion is growing again...

K: Is it difficult to proceed any longer?

W: This difficulty arises from my fear and anxiety...because I feel a great pressure to answer correctly...This pressure becomes a barrier in communication with the Voice...

K: I won't ask any more questions... You can tell me whatever comes to your mind...Relax and look around the room... You would see the things that are allowed for you to see...You can choose anything, without pressure, that can benefit people or that we need to learn... If you don't see or hear anything, you can rest... if they talk to you, you can listen at ease...

W: (in a solemn tone)... I love you... This is not the Voice of Wisdom speaking... I have a great amount of trust in you as a person, but you have shortcomings as well... (after being silent for a long period)... I wish you would instruct me to rest...

K: Relax and rest... let go all the images and pressure... rest in comfort...

W: (after resting about one minute)...Images are appearing before my eyes... But it is not easy to describe them with confidence...

K: You can tell me what you see... Look at them as they are...

W: (after a brief pause)...I see President ??? (name withheld by the author) ...of the United States... I'm being told many shed blood because of him ...This does not mean a war... it refers to a conspiracy... The United States will fall due to the evil it has committed... It has committed so many evil deeds... It will gradually lose internal control... Such loss will manifest physically and spiritually... There will come a movement to establish Black Republic... The Federation will collapse and smaller federations will rise... These smaller ones will not be disconnected from one another... It will become more loose state of federation over all... But some of them will have hostile relationship with others...

K: Will this happen in near future?

W: It is not so far... Each State will try to possess its own independent armed forces... (in a very strong tone)... The era of the United States is over ...I can assure you...

K: Is there another world scale war waiting for us?

W: Yes...

K: Which countries will be involved?

W: ...China will be out of it... (in a heavy dignified tone) ...This war is a must on our way to spiritual purification... You can say this is an organizing process of a civilization...

K: Is this what they refer to as Armageddon?

W: You can say that...

K: Is there a role for Korea in the war?

W: ...Korea will play a role after the war...

K: Will Korea fight in the war?

W: No.

K: Will it receive any damage from the war?

W: No... The United States and France will become adversaries to each other... Previous alliances will collapse and new alliances will form... It is not yet time to speak about in detail... (after a brief pause)... I see a piece of barley bread...

K: What does it mean?

W: I hear the Voices, but I don't understand what they mean... I cannot tune my frequency to the Voices...

K: Is the message too much for you?

W: Not really...

K: Are you feeling not well?

W: ...My stability has broken...

K: Shall I instruct you to rest more?

W: ...It won't do... I feel I can't do any more today... even with more rest...

K: Let's stop today, then...

W: Yes...

We both felt quite weighed down after completing the seventh session. We felt like we were given an overwhelming task because the message from the Voice was enough to get us in trouble if known to public as they were. The Voice told us to work together to get ready for the time to come. It told me to let the world know the messages but not for the fame or to satisfy intellectual curiosity in me, and it emphasized repeatedly, this young man must be protected. Won and I talked about these issues and decided to continue our work in a humble and open-handed manner. We decided to avoid asking any personal issue or question, and accept only what the Voice shows or tells us. We did not know how far this work will go, but we felt it also was not our decision to make.

What is the 'Akashic record'? Edgar Cayce, who was called a 'sleeping prophet', who delivered abundant information on mysterious subjects under hypnotic trance, cured difficult illnesses of many people, and produced countless prophecies, claimed all of his information came from 'Akashic Record'. He said all the information of the Universe is contained in it. I thought sages and prophets in history must have somehow extracted their wisdom and prophesies from this warehouse of information, and the Voice confirmed my supposition to be true.

I had a brother. He was three years younger than I, and we were always very close. As he grew as tall as I, we became more like best friends than brothers.

We pulled pranks on each other a lot, shared secrets and conversed deeply on various subjects. We understood and respected each other as close brothers should. Opposite from being aggressive, self-righteous and cynical as I am, he was gentle, generous and kind but never yielding when confronted injustice. His selfless character drew so many good friends around him. He often worried about my one-man army attitude and mercurial temperament. He joined Korean Army in 1982, as a member of graduate ROTC officers after graduating from Sogang University. He was 22 years old and his major was Economics and Management. After completing advanced military training as an officer in June the same year, he was given the rank of Second Lieutenant to be assigned as a platoon commander of the 21st Division of Army in Kangwon Province of Korea. He was in charge of guarding a sector of 155 mile long DMZ(Demilitarized zone) fence which divides South Korea from the North. He was always a caring leader who wrote frequently to me his concerns about his subordinates' safety and welfare, and about his lack of fear even in the most dangerous situations. He lamented and pitied the poor backgrounds and lack of high education among many of his platoon soldiers. In the early morning of 22nd September, 1982, I got a phone call from a staff officer of the 21st Division Headquarters. When I answered the call, he informed me, after a moment's uneasy hesitation, my brother was found dead with a gunshot wound on his head about half an hour ago at the mortar base of the platoon which was on a small hill. The staff officer was trying to paint the death as a suicide without any investigation or any tangible explanation. He even asked me 'Was there any family conflict at your home?' I answered coldly

'Watch your tongue. Are you insulting my family? We never had any such thing. How do you know, only after 30 minutes, it was suicide?' He stammered at my harsh response. 'Well...of course, we don't know for sure yet... anyway, we need family members here to take care of the matter.' So, my dear brother was found dead, after only three months on his duty at DMZ, with no witness and no apparent reasons, in very suspicious surroundings. In the late afternoon of the same day, my father and one of his close friend, and I arrived at the Division Headquarters.

Incredulous and dazed, we were guided to the place where the body of my brother was moved. I inspected his body, a rather deep and wide abrasive wound on the upper side of his face was apparent at first sight. A bullet hole was in the center of his forehead. The exit hole of the bullet was parallel to the inlet and was no wider or more damaged than the inlet. This finding didn't make sense to me because the outlet hole of a M-16 rifle shot on human body should be much bigger and extensively damaged than the inlet hole. And the trajectory of the bullet didn't make sense either. As the length of a M-16 rifle was about a meter long, to make a parallel trajectory of a bullet as I found on his head, the posture of the shooter should be very unnatural with muzzle fixed on his forehead and trigger finger far outstretched in front of his body. No one who tries to kill himself with a M-16 would choose this awkward and insecure posture to shoot. And another wound in the middle of his left shin caught my eyes, a deeply sunken fresh blue bruise as thick as a sole of the military boots. This meant only one thing. Someone facing my brother kicked him hard on the shin. The person must have been one of his superior officers because such a kick could be given only by the superiors of the victim. My father refused to sign on the paper which concluded the death as a suicide. The staff officers of the Division booked rooms for us at a motel in town for the procedures next morning.

At late night, when I was alone in deep grief, five of the Second Lieutenants of the 21st Division, who were all ROTC graduates and friends of my brother, visited me at the motel unexpectedly. They desperately appealed to me, some of them in tears, to investigate the death thoroughly. 'This is not a suicide. This can happen to any of us anytime. Please, to reclaim the honor of him and to protect us, we ask you to take all actions to start real investigation.' They said this and I promised them I will do whatever is needed. After returning home, I and my father filed petitions for reinvestigation at Army Crime Investigation Unit and Ministry of Defense. Both petitions were rejected immediately without any explanation. Unfortunately, the President of Korea at the time was a former General of the Army who took power under a martial law in the confusion after the assassination of the previous President who also was a former General of the Army. So, a request to re-examine a death in the Army fell to deaf ears of pro-military bureaucrats at the time. But my father finally abandoned to seek further petition only after he received a phone call from a stranger. He said to my father 'If you persist, your remaining son would suffer also.' Hence, my brother's death has become another questionable death in the suicide list of the Army record book, and all my family were deeply hurt and harbored inextinguishable anger and distrust toward the government. We could not accept his death as a suicide because he stated in one of his last letters to a friend 'To speak truth here is the same as I sign my own death sentence: A suicide by others.' Furthermore, his patrol roster of the night of his death was found in one of his pants pockets. If he planned to end his life early in the morning, he wouldn't have cared to write down the names of patrol members of the night, even less to carry the memo in his pocket. No one who knew him believed his death was a suicide. Waiting in the vain hope that the truth will be unveiled someday, so many years have passed. Although I had not said anything about my brother's death to Won before, the Voice answered my question and suggested me to let go of my spite and forgive those who are responsible.

Because I accept the theory of Karma and Transmigration, which states there are no coincidence in the world, and things happen for reasons, I thought I could forgive whoever shot my brother. They may enjoy a comfortable life for some time; I can calm myself in knowing they will eventually learn of their wrongdoing and suffer to pay for it. My brother also must have had a reason to leave the world so early as he did. As I know the souls who once became close in relationships meet repeatedly, I used to console myself in the firm belief that I'll meet him again. The Voice revealed my relationship to Won and suggested me to resolve my inner conflicts through these meetings. When I had chance to ask, I asked about what I have always been curious – Spirit or Demonic Possession.

For a psychiatrist, this phenomenon is an important issue. At times, patients with serious mental illness return to me worried after being told by a Shaman that they are possessed by evil spirits or a soul of a dead person. Bible also has references to demonic possession, and Buddhists frequently perform formal ceremonies to lead the wandering soul of a deceased person to heaven. If the existence of souls and spirits can be accepted, the possibility of their influences on living people should be studied also. I believe we should stop labeling this as mere superstition, and start investigation and open research instead. As a clinician who have witnessed and treated many so called Spirit Possessed patients, I agree to the Voice's explanation that Demonic Possession does not occur mostly by evil spirits, instead it occurs when one's negative and destructive energy attracts and amplify the similarly negative energy from the Universe. And whether it will come true or not, it was good to hear Korea will be spared from the future war and it will have an important role in the world after the war.

CHAPTER 9

The Eighth Meeting:

The Soul of Animals, Love, Secrets of Political leaders, UFO,
Causes of Mental Disease

(We did not regress to a past life in this eighth session).

K: Do you see anything?

W: ...I see the word 'Brandenburg'...

K: Anything else?

W: I don't see anything... I hear the words 'My beloved...' It says 'I love thee...' It is the Voice of an even higher being than what I used to hear... It tells me to embrace the Universe within me...

K: Does it mean 'Love'?

W: It feels more like another prophecy than love...

K: Let's enter the Third Room...

W: ...I entered the room... I feel other people have been here...

K: What are the things for you to see today?

W: The word 'Love' comes to my mind...

K: What does the room look like?

W: I can see the room, but all the views are symbolic... It looks like a library... There are many thick books, but they are not to be read with the eyes... they are there to save people from difficulties...

K: Do you hear the teaching on Love?

W: ...I don't hear any answers to it...

K: Shall I ask questions?

W: Yes...

K: Do animals have souls?

W: Animals have souls, but they differ from those of people... It is more like an instinctive action... The overall flow of Love is the same... the difference between the love in animals and that in people is... the love in animals is a tendency... It is an innate tendency which is driven by emotions of the animal... the Love which God desires is not this... God wants the kind of Love that builds through spiritual exchange between God himself and people... while you can call the Love in animals a relatively low one, the love from God is its highest form... The reason why you should practice such Love is... because Love is the starting point of Life... This means not only the sexual relationships or love among family members... As the primary current of the Universe is Love, you will be in tune with the pure energy of the Universe when Love is within you... Love is emphasized, not as much for the ones who are being loved, but because the souls of the ones who love make the pure energy of the Universe their own, and grow... One of the mysteries of

Love is that the one who loves acquires even greater strength which helps develop one's inner maturity and personal development... Love is not to confine, it is to open up... Most people love at the level of animal love, or love according to their innate tendency and survival instinct... The origin of the love for your own children or those who love you is your survival instinct... Under scrutiny, this cannot even be categorized as Love... However, such instinctual love can retain some of the life force that Love encompasses as well... Loving someone who loves you... or loving according to one's animalistic instinct, love that is led by emotions have the purpose of getting self satisfaction or profit in doing so... Many practice love with the purpose of their own survival... Ah...so many messages are pouring in at once... I don't know how to handle this... (after a brief pause)... When a man loves a woman without seeing her soul, the blind impulse to propagate offspring's becomes the motive... When someone loves you, why do you feel at ease and have desire to return the love? ...That's because it is based on the animalistic presumption that your life is not threatened by that person...It is always self-centered love... Why do parents wish their children to become better and achieve more? ...It is because they project their own wish-fulfillment onto their children... Why do people strive for higher office and worldly success? ...It is because they want to secure the base of their existence through such gains... But such forms of love cannot attain the fundamental power of Love of the Universe. ...The true Love lets everything thrive and grow...beyond one's own survival and preservation... Only when you practice such love, everything will finally become perfect... When you love only those who love you, others may get hurt in the process... because the right to survive of your beloved may precede that of others... You may even step on someone else's life to let your beloved survive... Yet, the law of the Universe does not allow one to violate other's lives... (in a strong and firm tone)...What you acquire from possession is merely phenomenal... The nature of the Truth is to enrich your soul by becoming free of negative energy within yourself through self-sacrifice, and by filling yourself with positive energy of the Universe... Those who practice animal love can give also... Such low level love can embrace and sacrifice as well... However, it is customary, momentary and seeks self-contentment in the end... The true Love is eternal and lets others prosper...It's brilliance getting stronger as time passes... Thus, when you love others, whether it be an erotic or agape one, you need to be sure of its motive... When love between a husband and wife is mainly of an erotic nature... It is, in fact, a self-satisfying love... It will eventually lead to disappointment toward each other... Because one needs to affirm and be affirmed of each other's survival territory, but this does not happen in a self-satisfying love... Such a couple eventually reaches the point where they can't coexist... Thus, the love between a couple which starts from Eros ends with confrontational discord... and to protect oneself from this discord, the couple sets an implicit truce and erects invisible boundary between each other... by not crossing the invisible lines between them, they think they have done their duties as partners... and become distant from each other... But when a husband and a wife love from the Universal point of view, they would be happy for the spiritual growth of each other... and they would stay in the middle of the positive energy current of the Universe... By emptying oneself willingly, one can infinitely expand the other's boundary... As the other comes into the emptied space of the one and expands, the energy of the Universe within one also expands with the other... The love between a husband and a wife, within the viewpoint of the Universe, unceasingly creates self-perpetuating process of love... Hence, one must fulfill one's self, always from the Universal viewpoint... When a couple practices such love... they will be able to love deeply without pretenses, hypocrisy or lies to avoid confrontation...and the respect for each other will grow as well... This means they will be filled with the positive energy of the Universe... It is the same with loving one's children...Do not treat your children in a self-satisfying fashion... (after a brief pause)... New messages are pouring into me, but I have become a little unstable to receive them...

K: Relax and rest a while...

W: (after resting about 30 seconds)... A husband and a wife must share sincere love... They may pretend not being hurt or dissatisfied by each other's actions and shortcomings, but such unresolved stresses accumulate. To protect themselves from further hurt, they hide their cold mind behind a smile... and the more smile one wears, more detached one becomes from the other... Such pretenses must be broken... Such pretenses are getting stronger with time, and they solidify as a cold knot of negative energy... This happens to all of you... Apply the principle of the Love of the Universe to your daily life... All the problems humankind have, including Karma, arises from self-obsession...

Won expressed a wish to relax and rest again at this point. The message after this rest was entirely different from the previous one.

W: ...Political leaders of the world felt about the fate which bounded them... John F Kennedy was much interested in spiritualism, and was not truly a Catholic... (after a pause)...Nikita Khrushchev and Kennedy had a secret entente...

K: Is it a secret to public?

W: (as if whispering) ...Yes...

K: What is it about?

W: Khrushchev had a need to consolidate his political base, and Kennedy was under pressure from the surreptitious power which drives United States... In order to strengthen their influences, they intended to prod the world into a state of tension and panic... Such was the ground of their mutual understanding... Khrushchev's thumping the floor of the UN building with his shoe was a premeditated political show...

K: What was the truth of Kennedy's death?

W: ...Since many groups were involved in his death, it is difficult to pinpoint who killed Kennedy... Oswald was merely a scapegoat... So many think they were benefited from the death of Kennedy...

K: Was the assassin from a conservative group?

W: Yes... they thought Kennedy had broken the promise he had made with them... Gandhi was aware that he would be killed... He did not know exactly who would assassinate him, but he had known about his own end... He was a Guru... a reincarnated Guru... Khrushchev grieved deeply when Kennedy died... The fact that Khrushchev was relieved from political power was a work of higher influence than this world... If he had stayed in power long enough... The United States might have disintegrated before the Soviet Union...

K: Was there a possible war between them?

W: No… The United States was structurally weaker than Soviet Union... It could have lost a competition of system...

K: What kind of person is Bill Clinton?

W: ...He is an aggregate of fabricated images... He can't do what he wants by himself ...you can say he is a puppet controlled by an organization ...(as if whispering)... He is really a pitiful person...

K: Was Kennedy killed because he had refused to do the puppet role?

W: All the Presidents of the United States since Kennedy... behaved cautiously...those who control the United States are not the Presidents, but the hidden characters behind them... This will not change just because the President is changed periodically... It is the system that is at fault... Many wars in the world are controlled by these people behind the scene...I see the word 'Trust'...and number '250' ...I also see people walking in New York City... The Voice says 'Kim Dae-jung' will become the next president of South Korea, but I can't be sure...(He was retired from active politics at the time.)... I see the word that the next President of South Korea will be Kim Dae-jung... But I am afraid to say so for sure...

K: What kind of person is he?

W: A cunning man... but he is not lacking in leading a country...

K: What can you say about the current President of South Korea?

W: He is a man of strong will-power, but there are many differences between his public persona and private side ...(after a pause of about half a minute)... I feel there is no more talk of politics...

K: Relax and rest as long as you need... Erase all the images from your mind and just relax... (after a few minutes, he resumed talking)

W: ...India's intention to use nuclear weapons on Pakistan must be stopped...

K: Do they really intend to use it?

W: The probability is dangerously high...

K: How is the relationship between China and Taiwan?

W: War will not break out between the two... If there had to be a war, it would be restricted to a regional skirmish...Deng Xiaoping's death is not far away... I see a name 'Quiao Shih' ...Jiang Zemin's political power is not secure enough...

K: Is it possible for Quiao Shih to become the successor of Deng?

W: Yes... but if he succeeds... it will be a takeover with force... If Jiang Zemin rules, China will stay as one nation, but it will become two separate entities if Quiao Shih rules...

K: How will it divide?

W: It will divide into North China and South China...

K: What will be the relationship between the two Chinas?

W: It will become an adverse relationship... South China will be ruled by a Shanghai faction, and North China will be ruled by a Beijing faction... I feel North China will crumble first...

K: What will become the future of India?

W: ...It is very bright... It will become one of the leading nations of the world...

K: Will their spiritual energy play a role in the future?

W: It may shrink... but it can't be overlooked.

K: Are there other life forms in the Universe and can we be born into their worlds?

W: (in a solemn tone)...It is not yet the time to talk about the subject...

K: Do UFOs physically exist?

W: Yes...but it is not yet time to discuss it...

K: Is there a cure for those chronic schizophrenics who resist all the current medical treatments available?

W: There are a few causes why people suffer from mental illness... I'll tell you two main causes... First, the functions of mental and neural system can get damaged by the use of excessive energy... Second, one may suffer mental illness due to evil spirits... Many of those who cannot be helped are more often ill due to evil spirits; otherwise, it is due to the irreversible damage of the nervous system in the patient's brain... Excessive use of mental energy can physically destroy the microscopic connecting points of nerve cells in our body... This is similar to an electric wire get overloaded and burn away to break when excessive electricity is connected to it... Damage at the connecting points, so called synapses, cannot be restored for now... But, in the future, Medicine will be able to repair such damages... Many symptoms of mental patients are also developed as a self-defense mechanism... When Medicine can develop a treatment which can open their closed minds, they will be cured... Controlling the vibration frequency of the body, about which I mentioned before, also will cure what's impossible to cure now...

K: Is there any treatment for cases of strong evil spirits taking control of patients?

W: The only way to expel such evil spirits... is Love...

K: Do patients have ability to practice such love?

W: (firmly)...No...

K: Is it Love from those around the patient?

W: (strongly)...Yes, it will be possible when Positive energy drives out Negative one.

K: Do you mean the love and devotion of the patient's family and doctor?

W: No, it is not such love... Only the Love that contains the Truth of the Universe makes it possible...

K: Are there people who can provide such Love?

W: Yes... as Jesus did so, those who lead such a life can do it...

K: Do such people exist?

W: They are hidden now, but will be revealed...

K: Why do you teach us all these things?

W: ...We wish people to change...and to prepare for the coming age...

K: Are we the ones who fit your purpose?

W: You will fit as much as you open your mind...

K: What does it mean to pursue Psychicism

W: ...Most of those who pursue Psychicism become dominated by evil spirits... They often see illusions... What I say 'Illusions' does not mean 'un-realistic images', I mean 'evil spirits'. There are many instances where evil spirits appear in various disguises... (firmly)... There is no Truth in such appearances... The biggest blind spot of psychicism is... it lacks Love... In order to retain the fundamental energy of the Universe, Love of highest level is essential... It can be called 'Mercy' as well... Without it, the pursuit of spiritual phenomena itself can lead to self-destruction...

K: Do you mean such study can elicit evil spirits to influence the student?

W: (in a strong tone) ...Yes... evil spirits can have great energy... The difference between evil spirits and good ones, is whether they have the ultimate Love of souls or not... And what you need to know in this chaotic age is, even evil spirits can appear in the shape of love... To distinguish evil from good, you need to live a life of Love yourself... Without living such a life, you cannot tell the difference between hypocritical love and real love... You cannot practice Love in theory, nor is it attained by being taught. It happens only when you live it...

K: Is it possible to meet the soul of loved one who deceased?

W: It is better not to attempt...

K: Is it meaningless to do?

W: Yes...it only makes people confused further.

K: What about hypnotic Past-Life Regression Therapy?

W: ...It is a very delicate issue... There is no good or evil in the technique itself... though, depending on the user, it can turn out to be good technique or an evil one... When a therapist with goodness uses the method, it becomes a good method... But if one with evil intention practices it, it will turn out evil... The beginning of both will look similar though...

K: Is it only meaningful when practiced with love and intention to help the patient?

W: You can say so... but no therapist is perfect, as everyone is partial... There is no one who is complete... It is important to remember you are always insufficient in some way... you should be humble...There hasn't been a complete person yet... I must rest...

K: Relax deeply and rest... clear all the images and message from your mind...

W: (after resting about 20 seconds)... I see a scoop... but I can't tell the meaning of the image... We should stop here today...

Won entered the room of 'Akashic Record' as he did last time without regressing into his past life memories. The messages we heard in the room were entirely at the discretion of the Voices, but they kindly answered many of my questions. Do animals have souls? It is a question asked by many, including animal lovers. I also know from experience we can develop spiritual connection with beloved animals. Who can possibly refuse to smile at the excitement of a puppy greeting its owner's return home? Moreover, the theory of transmigration from ancient times has claimed that humans can be reborn as animals in their next life. And there are people who believe human souls must have once resided in the body of animals in the long process of soul's growth toward enlightenment and perfection. I once read with interest the autobiography of Yogananda, a famous Yogi from India. A story in the book showed me even animal souls advance in their own way. One day, young disciples of Yogananda found their beloved fawn nearly dead from a mortal disease. They requested their teacher to pray for the fawn not to die. Unable to deny his young disciples' heart-felt petition, he started long and sincere prayer. After a while, the fawn seemed to recover from its illness. But when Yogananda dozed off briefly during the long and exhausting prayer, the soul of the fawn appeared in his dream and pleaded with him in tears, 'I must leave now to advance another step, Please do not hold me back here.' From this incident, he stated, he realized everything has its own time, and we must not seek anything out of our self-centered viewpoint. Can people be born as animals in their next life? The Voice told us the difference between the soul of human and that of animal. Even the lowest soul of a person is higher than the soul of an animal, as it is in sym-pathy with God, the Voice said. The idea of being reborn as an animal in the next life because of one's wrongdoing can be understood as a metaphor. To be born as a pig in the next life may mean the person will have pig-like tendency, and to be born as a dog means having dog like traits.

But, can people really be born as animals in their next life? I have come to my conclusion after having many hundreds of patient cases of Past-Life Regression and extensive research on the subject. If a person degenerates one life after another, he will eventually be born as a person with many serious flaws and pains. In this way, he will repay his errors according to the law of Karma, and restart the process of advancement of his soul from then on.

The Voice told us in a part of the dialogue which I didn't include in this book, the soul of a person is made differently from that of an animal from the outset, and it clearly stated that we don't need to be concerned about the transmigration of animals as they are not affected by same Karma as humans'. Furthermore, reincarnation in the form of an animal as in Buddhist teaching is only symbolic and metaphoric to emphasize the importance of moralistic life. And if, under hypnosis, one sees oneself as an animal in a past life, the Voice explained, it is not real life memories but a symbolic representation of the life one experienced. Although almost all the memories as human beings in past lives are real ones, the Voice said, one may rarely see a life of symbolic fabrication as well. But an experienced therapist will be able to distinguish the actual life memories from the fabricated one. Let's have a look at Hindu teachings on reincarnation as an animal, the ancient Manu scripture or Manusmrti states 'A rational soul or higher-than-animal principles does not reincarnate in the body of an animal. Those who have not realized sacred principles are born into a lowly body because they neglected their duties while buried in sensual desires.' It seems some people reincarnate as humans with certain mental traits or characteristics of certain types of animal. For instance, a sly personality is represented as a snake, while greediness as a swine. I personally have not seen a patient who, among many hundreds, remembered a past life as an animal, nor have I heard of such reports in numerous cases of past life regression from abroad. Teaching of the difference between love in animals and the Love of the Universe answers many aspects of our relations with emotionally close people. When this teaching is applied, various encounters in our life that seed Joy, sorrow, hatred and despair in us also can be understood. All the human relations we experience in life- parents and siblings, spouses, children, friends and coworkers, and enemies- also can be understood when this teaching from the Voice is applied. Though unfortunate encounters may tire and sadden our lives to the limit, we have no way to avoid all those painful encounters. The Voice tells us to love all these encounters in a non self-satisfying manner, and those who love will become more mature and happier than those who are being loved. How many newlyweds leave on their honey moon, radiating happiness from their faces, in the dream of long waited moments of happiness will spread before their eyes forever from now on? Yet, reality soon wears the couple down as days go by, leaving both of them exhausted to be negligent and indifferent to each other. Eventually many couples become estranged in this way to live as almost strangers under a same roof. Blaming each other cannot solve anything. For whatever the reason, there are many who choose the wrong person as their life-long partner. 'I must have been blind to marry such a woman.' I'll be OK as soon as he dies.' 'I am living with him only because of my children.'

A psychiatrist is a person who has to listen to such laments several times a day. It is true there are wives and husbands who are abused unilaterally by the other, but in most cases, the abuse is mutual. Reason for this is, people get disappointed, even grow hatred when their partners do not cooperate fully with their selfish desires. Why does a romantic and innocent couple transform into self-centered and greedy people after marriage, occupied only in increasing material wealth and worldly success? Materialism not only planted obsession with material goods in our minds, but also created greediness and possessiveness toward everything and everyone around us. When we wish to possess other's love and devotion as we possess material wealth and social status, the frustration and despair begin as they are not attainable materials. When a couple's goal in marriage becomes to buy a grand house, accumulate wealth to live materially better than others, their children will be trained in the same competitive and covetous way. Forsaking greed seems to be an impossible task in human level consciousness. Who would abandon self-interest, and love others as themselves when there is no proof of such behavior is better for us? To teach us how transient and meaningless is greed or obsession; unavoidable misfortunes and disasters ambush us in the course of our lives. They are the real teachers of Truth. In a split second, they steal from our bosom, the most precious that once seemed to be ours. Greed and envy will lose its ground when people realize the fact that possessing material goods does not mean much. We may feel more content when given more, but such content will not be appealing enough to become the goal of life itself. Selfless Love of the Universe may be possible only after we experience many disappointments in life and overcome them successfully.

Overcoming the disappointments and starting afresh to find an everlasting, unchanging value of life, we meet again the Love and the Truth. Love of the Universe is the same as what Jesus taught in 'Love thy neighbor.' and

Buddha's emphasis on 'mercy'. These teachings can be misunderstood or interpreted in self righteous way when taught in the frame of religion. Yet, it is not the fault of the teaching, the artificial system we call religion is at fault. Though a religion basically teaches enlightenment and good deeds, it has flaws and limitations as it was created by human minds. But, to teach large group of people together and develop support system among them, building an organization like religion is inevitable. However, the weakest point of an organization is that its maintenance can become its primary purpose. In the efforts to keep the organization intact, the original purpose of it can weaken to be replaced by the survival of the organization. Today, many people hesitate to take part in a religion. Although they acknowledge the noble teachings of religions, people disapprove the long history of arrogance and self-righteous attitude of religions. Religious figures who act as if they have monopolized the Truth also drive away people from joining religions.

On top of these, the increasing number of hypocritical pseudo-believers who speak beautiful words of faith, but live a life of a non-believer, are discouraging people to join a religion. When people attend religious ceremony to make business contacts or to befriend influential ones, churches and temples will become places for social gathering, not places to attain true freedom through spiritual growth.

How can we develop respect and trust toward religion when we see hypocrisy and corruption in the people who practice religion? Where can people turn to when they cannot find love and peace even in religions? The answers are plainly to be seen in many problems of our society. Money gets thicker than blood, and the number of irresponsible people who cannot understand and overcome their frustrations is increasing, to harass others for their own misery. The root cause of all the pathological phenomena in human society is 'Unhappy people'. I cannot agree more to the teaching of the Voice, 'The Love of the Universe has the power to resolve obstacles to the Truth and happy life.' I have no intention to discuss the authenticity of the Voice's words on the secretive dealings of the world leaders and prophecies of the future, because I can't prove or disprove them for now. Still, they sound highly probable when we view situations mentioned with common sense. I have decided to believe the information given by the Voice for two reasons. First, there is no reason why Won can't possess the ability which Edgar Cayce and Paul Solomon had when hypnotized. Second, to my judgment, as the teachings of the Voice are very moving and enlightening in all subjects other than unverifiable prophecies, I don't see any reason why it would lie or fabricate to mislead us. Nonetheless, as the future is not yet set like the past, I think it would be better not to be obsessed with the prophecies of the future. A big part of the assassination of Kennedy is still veiled. The investigation report itself had been classified as a top secret, and the evidences and testimonies against the known conclusion- 'Oswald shot Kennedy'- were hastily discarded. Compared to the normal legal procedures of the United States which deliberately take long time to conduct a complete investigation, the case of Oswald in relation to Kennedy's death seems rather bizarre. Gandhi was a person of different class than most other political leaders. The whole world was moved by his saint-like nature. Albert Einstein commented upon hearing Gandhi's death. 'Our descendants won't believe the fact that such a great man once existed.' If Gandhi had been a reincarnated Guru, we may better understand the source of his immense spiritual strength. His grand-daughter testified once that Gandhi had her to bring him all the important documents in the morning of his death, saying 'I must sign them all today, for there will be no tomorrow.' He perhaps had known about his assassination as a Guru might. Although I did not disclose them in this book, the Voice also told us other secrets. They include, among other things, the secret surroundings of the death of Mao Zedong, the death of Marilyn Monroe and the power behind it, the death of Kim Ilsung -the former leader of North Korea, and the secrets of present political leaders of South Korea. About Psychics, the Voice gave me answer to my question 'Where does this ability come from?' The answers given were the same as what I always thought. I have been curious about the reality of Psychicism for long time. The hidden science of mysterious phenomena of spiritual realm always appealed to me as a subject I must tackle someday. Years ago, I met a man who wrote quite a few books on Psychicism. He claimed in his books that most diseases are caused by evil spirits and they can be healed by the method he developed.

Although I didn't believe his claims, I was curious about the grounds of such a bold assertion. If his method could help even one patient, it would not be an attitude of a scientist to ignore what he had to say without a look at the evidence he offers. The first impression I got when I met the man was 'He is very intelligent.' He laid out before me his theories and achievements. Even though he had some believable theories and claims, I was disappointed. He was full of airs and was fascinated and immersed in his own claims. He talked about 'The highest god' in the spiritual world as if he was bragging about a powerful friend who listens to all his requests. He also boasted that the highest god thanked him very much when he corrected a mistake of the god, a mistake the god hadn't been aware of. I decided the man was lacking truth or sanity and walked away from him. When a huge obstacle, seemingly impossible to solve or overcome, confronts us, we often feel temptation to get some help from divination or a fortune teller. Some of my patients talk about such experiences as well. But I never saw a patient who really resolved his obstacle in such a manner. Many people with simple anxiety are being diagnosed as spirit possession by shamans or religious healers to waste huge sum of money on prayers, talisman or various forms of exorcism. But, their symptoms usually get better only after resuming appropriate psychiatric treatment. Even if someone claims to possess a supernatural power to heal others, as such power is not easy to verify objectively, there remains certain amount of danger in seeking help from such a person. The Voice emphasized that it is perilous to pursue the spiritual world without good intention and love within oneself. It told me that our interest and curiosity can attract undesirable spirits to us and we can become controlled by them. In hypnosis, people's consciousness expands to cover the areas normally inaccessible when in superficial consciousness. Memories of fetus state, Past-lives, In-between life period all fall into this category. By exploring these memories, we can discover sources and the relations of symptoms and problems of patients.

As I have seen so many difficult patients get better or healed by this approach, I have come to accept the validity of their memories. But, whether the memories of those periods are real or not is a serious scientific question. We will have more space to look into the matter in other part of this book. I believe psychiatrists must study and research the Past-Life regression therapy, because it has a very strong therapeutic effect when used on some patients who could get little help from other conventional therapies. As psychiatry should be different from other medical fields that only focus on the material aspects of human being, the realm of modern psychiatry should grow wider and deeper to encompass all the Transpersonal and Transcendental experiences of people. In Past-life regressions, patients often recognize familiar faces from their current life and explain away the meanings of each life in their own interpretation. When considering all these unusual phenomena in hypnosis, we can postulate that the one who recalls those memories is the patient's soul itself. It seems to me that the words 'subconsciousness', 'superconsciousness' and 'soul' are interchangeable in practical sense. If we accept this concept, it will be easier to understand why spiritual phenomena occur more frequently in hypnosis, the state which our subconscious rules. If a therapist with evil intention regresses a patient into past lives could it be possible that the therapist's negative energy would attract the interference from evil spirits? When I asked this question to the Voice, it gave me an answer of great significance. It answered that a good intention and a right self-consciousness are the most important qualities for the therapist. I was also told, 'You can practice the technique, but only when necessary after a careful consideration.' I have found that the initial reactions of patients after experiencing their first past-life regression are largely the same. They come out of hypnosis shaken but skeptical, 'Can this not be a fabrication of my mind?' they ask me as well as to themselves. However, passing time and the repeating regressions encourage their faith to deepen and increase the understanding of the therapy. Especially, the memory of death scenes and what comes after it are so impressive; they find it similar to the testimonies of those who have undergone a Near-Death-Experience. As a result of these experiences, the fear of death becomes reduced in them, and they begin to see their life as something meaningful and eternal. The symptoms and problems of theirs usually lessen and disappear, some immediately and some gradually, during this process. As we already saw, Won resolved his ill feelings toward China immediately after his first session. The reason why patients have no choice but to accept the recovered memories as their own in time, is because the memory itself is so persuasive. Though some memories are very vivid and others are vague and indistinct, they all include very persuasive and appealing clues to their current problems. Patients can't simply dismiss the memories as creations of their imagination because what they haven't even thought about appears to them as memories of highly personal nature, accompanied by strong emotion which befits the situations in their memory. Many similarities are felt between the past and the present, including personal traits, talents and relationships with those around the patient. As some memories can be painful and disturbing to the patient, the therapist should provide warm and considerate guidance and protection. An important role of a therapist is to help patients to experience their memories comfortably no matter how intense emotions accompany them. Inexperienced therapists might not know the importance of this aspect, to push too hard or lead too eagerly to cause stresses in patients. Therefore, I think only the therapists with extensive experience in other forms of hypno-therapy should attempt the Past-Life regression therapy. Another important aspect we must be aware of, is that the psychiatric principles and psychological interpretations are also needed in analyzing and interpreting the past-life memory. Consequently, therapists with professional knowledge and experience in psychiatric treatment are the ones who can qualify to practice past-life regression therapy. At times, as past-life regression patients need medication, who else other than psychiatrists can be more qualified? Though the Voices denied any answer to the questions regarding other life forms in the Universe, they acknowledged the existence of UFOs. Although they declined to discuss the subject further, my impression was that they would reveal more when the right time comes. I also asked about Chronic Schizophrenia, which frustrates psychiatrists more than any other disease. 'Destroyed nervous system and the work of evil spirits are the main causes and they will be overcome in the future' was the answer.

I think, many readers will feel uneasiness by my repeated mentioning of evil spirits. I myself don't feel comfortable using such words. Yet, I believe it is not right to ignore the possible existence of evil spirits just because we don't like the idea. In fact, I asked the Voice with a hope that such evil spirits didn't exist. However, the answer was the opposite of my hope. As I can't ignore this answer, I feel I need to study and investigate this issue further and other scientists should do the same.

CHAPTER 10

The Ninth Meeting:

Life in Egypt, Hell, Love and Modesty, Self-content, Increase in population, Teachings on Judgment

(In the ninth session, Won regressed into another past-life).

K: Where are you?

W: In Egypt...

K: Are you alone?

W: ...I am not sure...

K: What are you doing?

W: ...Supervising a construction site...maybe a pyramid is being built... It's not clear.

K: Relax and go deeper into hypnosis... You will see clearly in time...

W: ...I am a foreman who controls laborers...

K: Will you describe your appearances?

W: I am 180 – 190 centimeters tall and... about 40 years of age... I beat a laborer severely once... and he is my superior at office in this life who has harassed me much recently...

K: The one who got beaten by you is now your superior at work?

W: Yes... I have debt to repay him...

K: What is your name?

W: ...Orakente ...is all I can remember...

K: Orakente?

W: Yes... I think I came from Ethiopea.

K: Do you have dark skin?

W: ...Fairly dark...

K: When is this?

W: ...It is about 4th Century B.C.

K: Who is the Pharaoh at the time?

W: ...I think there are aristocrats... not Pharaoh...

K: Do the aristocrats rule?

W: ...We are not building a tomb for a Pharaoh... but constructing a private building for an aristocrat...

K: What kind of a construction is it?

W: ...It maybe we are building a palace or a mansion...

K: Do you have any particular trade?

W: No... I don't... I am a very cunning man... but I don't occupy a high position... I am a person who bullies my inferiors and flatters my superiors...

K: Tell me about your family.

W: I have a wife... she is very passive... I have a lover other than my wife... I do not wish to lose either of them... I am not family-oriented, nor do I have much affection for my lover either... I am rather violent in nature...

K: What are your feelings when you supervise the work site?

W: I always wish to complete the construction earlier by slave-driving the workers...

K: What type of building are you constructing now?

W: ...I see columns similar to those in Greek temples... It maybe a library... It is in Alexandria... Those who are in power now are not originally from Egypt...

K: Where did they come from?

W: ...From Greek regions...

K: Do Greeks rule the place?

W: ...They have the power, but they are the ones who are assimilated to the culture of Egypt... Their ancestors were Greeks, but they are the same as natives of this country...

K: Let's go to the next important scene...

W: ...I have amassed a small fortune by tricking my superiors, I was not poor... but I have built much resentment about my social status... Once, a man told me not to live the way I did... But I ignored his advice... I had a desire to live like a nobleman... I was a very aggressive man... I hear someone telling me, 'do not be afraid to give.'

K: Is the Voice telling you?

W: Yes...

K: Let's proceed to the moment of your death...

W: ...I am stabbed to death...

K: How old are you?

W: ...Forty one or two years old...

K: Who killed you?

W: There was a man who I abused much...He took his revenge on me... I see my superior at work in this life that has vexed me much...

K: Do you still have a problem with your superior in this life?

W: Yes... But, I try hard not to hate him...

K: Did the man confront you with a knife?

W: No... He ambushed me from behind...

K: Have you passed the moment of death?

W: I am watching the death scene...calmly... I had difficulty in breathing as his knife pierced through my right lung... He also stabbed my back several times...

K: What had you done to him?

W: I whipped him severely and seized his assets... as well as his daughter... I did not feel guilty about such actions because they were rather common things at the time...

K: He must have suffered much by you.

W: Yes... That's why he waited for the chance to kill me... I hear the words, 'When you die...' I think it is a message but I am not sure what it means...

K: What happened after you died?

W: ...It was very agonizing... after death...

K: Where did you go after death?

W: ...I was whipped...

K: Where were you whipped?

W: ...You can say it is Hell... I was punished much more than I did to others...

K: Have you learned anything while being tormented there?

W: ...I don't know for sure... I could only think of pain at the time...

K: What were the lessons of that life?

W: ...I learned not to try to possess too much... I had to learn to be content with what I had... I hear some other words, but I am not sure...

K: Relax and rest awhile... Erase all the images from your mind... (I told him to rest for awhile)...

While resting, Won said, 'Various images are passing by, but I can't pick out any particular message from the Voice. I cannot relax completely...' I woke him from hypnosis at this report, then guided again into deeper hypnosis.

K: Relax completely, do not try too hard to see or hear anything...

W: ...Through the history, the causes of social change start from mixture of the wish to confirm one's existence, desire to secure one's life and the instinct to be protected from others... All the social changes, including revolution and reformation, start from the desire to protect one's living condition and to expand one's life territory... Yet, the reasons why people have never truly succeeded in revolutions are, first, their revolutions began from an egotistical point of view, second, they never were truly aware of the meaning of the True Change... Even though liberal democracy of Western Europe and social democracy of Northern European countries may have provided much materialistic benefit to many... this is a deceptive strategy which the ones in power have hypocritically offered to secure their positions... Reformation plans and ideologies from such an authority eventually lead to even deeper corruption to bring more pain to the people of the opposite side... So called social reformations, so far, are only a zero-sum game. In other words, such reformations have only brought security of the society from the sacrifice of one side... However, the people who have benefited through such a materialistic social system are not much satisfied, because humans are spiritual beings. Materialistic social security cannot fulfill the spiritual side of people... True Revolution, True Life is not a gathering of selfish people... It is possible only when people have the faith that they will be protected by a higher being even if they sacrifice themselves by stepping out of their protective shelter and abandon their possessions... only when such faith spreads, can a revolution succeed... Sharing such faith is more important than reforming a social system...Therefore, a true social change can happen when people focus more on sharing altruistic attitude, or learn the mind of God than being obsessed with social reform itself... Look, throughout history, people have not enjoyed contented lives... They have amended and added many articles of law, changed systems and organizations to achieve security of their lives and the society they live in... But, nothing fundamental has changed yet... Only the forms and shapes of authority and possession changed... But as the authority and possession are only illusions, those who once held them dear face even deeper emptiness at the end... Even the most reliable things in human society- wealth, knowledge, systems cannot give ultimate answers as they have their own limitations... Now is the time you must take a new point of view... Instead of desiring grand things and ideas, you must train yourselves to begin sharing small things...What is needed is always provided to those who pursue a soul and heaven... A true social change will take place only when you share and embrace many within your own sphere, not being obsessed with keeping your domain to yourself... Message ends here...

K: Relax...

W: ...The Voice talks again... about the difference between men and women... It says 'A man enjoys happiness in ownership,' and 'a woman enjoys happiness in confirmation.' What the Voice means by 'happiness' is 'satisfaction'. And it says that people cannot be satisfied because men constantly attempt to possess and women want to confirm endlessly... I hear another message... A solution to this problem... But the message is like a ball of entangled yarn... I cannot untangle it...

(I let him relax and rest for a short time and proceeded again).

W: ...I hear words... 'Cultivate your capacity to contain other's minds'... The Voices encourage us to do this... 'Not only understand other's positions, but also the happiness and sadness of other's should become mine as well... Resonance in emotions solicits resonance of souls... and resonance in souls brings resonance in emotions... Thus, many people, no matter what type of people they are, search for love that can bring resonance in their souls... Consoling others and sharing true love is not possible with sympathy alone... Resonance of soul must be added to it to achieve such tasks... Leaders in the future should be people who can match their soul's resonance to the resonance of emotions of people... They should be able to share and modulate such ability with masses... Things will be different in the future... The world which has been ruled by power, talent, and ability so far will become to be ruled by the people who can share resonance of souls together... Such people have increased in numbers... From now on, the society will be divided into two large groups of people. One will be those who become more corrupt in material pursuit, and the other will be the people who seek maturity and purity of their souls...

K: Two extreme opposite groups of people will be formed?

W: Yes... The pure ones will become even purer... and corrupt ones will become more corrupt...However, people will not call the corruption as 'corruption'... They will call it a 'general tendency' of people... But, as we mentioned before, those who do not resonate with the flow of the Universe will perish... The might of a man is not made of talents he has... It comes from the capacity of his soul which can resonate with the Universe, the Mind of God... Strive to cultivate the capacity of your soul... If a part of your soul can not resonate with other people, strive to achieve the resonance with them... If your endeavor is not fruitful, then, seek it in prayer... Jesus once said: 'Thou shall not enter the gate of heaven without first becoming like a child'... because the souls of children are easy to resonate... Shed many tears, and do not fear to lose your face... To human eyes, the phenomenon of soul's resonance may appear inferior to see... Yet, such an appearance will eventually overcome other apparently superior forms... The weak triumphs over the strong... (in a slow but strong tone)...What is truly strong appears as weak...

K: (after a long silence)... Any other message?

W: Nervousness and palpitation, I feel inside of me... My stability broke when the telephone rang outside a while ago... My heart has been thumping loudly since then...

I led him to relax once again and we rested about half a minute. When I tried to proceed again, he said, 'I am afraid and nervous because I have a strong sense of duty to deliver the message correctly, but the message is being given to me as large clumps of information. My stability is being broken as I try too hard to relay the message correctly... To relieve his tension, I said following words, "We have much time... We have much future... We will know what we need to know... Don't be too eager to receive the entire message... When you become too eager, you become obsessed and your stability will break... You will get message correctly when your mind is calm and smooth like a mirror surface... Obsession and eagerness cannot unscramble all the incoming messages...Relax and just watch what is being given to you..."

'Tell me to go deeper.' Won asked me. As I guided him deeper as he requested, we heard the Voices again.

W: Do you know about 'Icarus'?

K: Yes... Go ahead...

W: I see a picture... and the word 'Icarus'... I see him from Greek Mythology, he who tried to fly with bird's feathers attached to him... I hear the Voices saying many people are becoming like an Icarus in the realm of spirit...

K: Do you mean people have false belief that they can understand spirits with logic?

W: You are free to arrange feathers and attach them to yourself, but when you try to fly with this arrangement, you will surely fall ...Where should your action stop? ...You must stop at the point of collecting feathers... Many fail eventually because they do not know about this... Therefore, a man can possess the truth and proceed to the secrets of the Universe, only when he clearly realizes the foundation of his existence... There are two or three types of people who fail... People who think themselves as God approach sun in that illusion and melt themselves down. Another group follows the false image of God, not real one, to stray away from the truth and cling to self- satisfactory faith... They are the ones who are over-confident in human talents and decorate themselves with seemingly righteous morality... (in a solemn and strong tone)... Both of these types will fail in the end... We must realize that all souls are created by God, and our lives are shared by God... All life can become a part of God... Therefore, we may appear to possess ability and shape similar to God... But, we must clearly understand the limit here...When you think you are God, the flow from the Universe to you gets blocked... Following distorted image of God and Truth also sever the connection to the Universe... Thus, being overconfident... Messages are becoming blurred... I am in too shallow a state...

I guided him into deeper relaxation and proceeded again. He jumped to another message without finishing the previous one.

W: The Voices say, 'When you see the fecal remains of an elephant, you can tell the status of the elephant... A big person leaves big marks, and a small person leaves small marks... You must observe the trace of a man when evaluating him... Without being hasty, you must observe patiently the marks of his soul... Many things in the world are getting contaminated... Many people try to embellish their marks through false images and information, but, with time, such marks will eventually rot away without any trace, just like fecal remains dry, rot and decompose into nothing...Dung of an elephant belongs only to the elephant...and the existence of the elephant is not erased even though it's dung rot away under the blazing sun...' The Voices are telling me the meaning of this message... When an elephant drops its dung, it becomes an indication to people that an elephant has passed... Even though the dung itself dries up and crumbles into nothing under the heat of sun... The important thing is the existence of the elephant... It does not change into nothing... Can a small animal become an elephant by gathering large amounts of its fecal matter into the size and shape of an elephant dung?... Even if a man builds a mountain of false images that are not his own and presents products that are not his own making... They will become meaningless when they decompose in time... In other words, what is important is the fact that the elephant exists... The message is being delivered to me in big clumps... Perhaps, I should relay it with more caution in selecting words... When evaluating a man, you get to know him better by observing his actions, but the impressions he made in us fade away as time flows...but, if the man continues to exist, he will continue to leave impressions in us... Even though we forget them, new impressions will keep accumulating in us... In short, it is not the action of the man that matters, it is his existence that matters... If the man possesses a soul that is capable of producing great impressions in us... the fact that he exists among us is enough, regardless of whether we remember or forget the impressions made by the man...

Some people produce false images, as if they possess souls of goodness, to protect themselves and hide their shameful doings... But, when they fade in our memory, even the traces of their existence disappear along with them... Thus, we should avoid building false images of ourselves to prevent the emptiness which results from them... Instead, we should try hard to uplift our souls to such a high level...

Praise, fame, good deeds... Many will regard you highly when you enjoy these things... But they produce even more emptiness in you if you don't have a matching soul to go with them... Hence, you are not to deceive yourself... Build more capacity in your soul that can contain the fruits of the Truth... Please, focus on this task... Do not remember the achievements of your actions...An elephant steps forward without remembering its excrement... But people will become amazed of the presence of the elephant by seeing its droppings... It is the same with us... We must not focus on our good qualities or the results of our good deeds...When we concern ourselves with them, we produce false images... When you have a soul of big capacity, people will know you correctly by seeing your traces...

But, if you build images without becoming like them yourself, people may follow you at the beginning... However... they would not be able to find the source of those images... because there is only a dung beetle instead of an elephant... Though many expected to see an elephant, they find only a dung beetle in the end... In their frantic search for the elephant, people would crush the dung beetle dead under their feet... So many people are busy pursuing false images, try to produce beyond their capacity, and hide behind masks...to end up being stepped on... Indeed, we must build up our soul's capacity first... We must become an elephant first... Are you an elephant, or a dung beetle? ...A dung beetle may live long by building a small heap of dung... When the beetle makes its dung heap too large... It attracts people who are searching for an elephant, and the beetle will be squashed under their feet... I see the image of frogs... When frogs balloon up their throats to their limit and croak loudly, the collective sound may shake even a mountain... but those who know about the frogs are not afraid of the sound, nor are they interested in the frogs themselves... Yet, people who don't know about frogs become curious, and they will be disappointed when they find the source of the sound... They would even lose the interest they initially had... Many frog-like people try to croak much louder than a frog might... They may be content with the unnatural loudness of the sound... the listeners know that it is the sound of a frog... Many politicians are like such frogs... but, not only are those who want to seize the power of the world frogs... Look into yourself... Isn't there a frog within you? ...Isn't there a dung beetle within you? ...We must remove the froth from our lives... We must eliminate the foam of our soul... No one will accuse or scorn you because you reveal the true shape of yourself... On the contrary, they will feel embarrassed before you...This is because everyone in this world is a frog or a dung beetle... Many men of cloth are dung beetles hiding behind elephant masks... They may believe themselves as tigers, for their sound shakes a mountain, they are only frogs... Many forget this fact to end up tearing their throats to shreds in the foolish attempt to croak louder...You must find yourself... You must uncover yourself... Only those who have found themselves know where to go...and how to find the direction... A man is not the God... and he cannot become the God by his endeavor... Message ends here... You may ask questions...

K: Do our souls mature only through loving others' souls?

W: ...You can say it is mutual relationship... Neither part is dependent on the other... When we love, we grow... and when we grow, we love... There is a tool we can use to measure the degree of love... It is 'Modesty'... Having modesty does not mean to degrade you. It means you accept other's existence as it is... What is modesty? ...Is it modesty when a father bows to his son? ...Is it merely bowing your head to other person? ...It is not so ...You may bow your head to your parents, but you can acknowledge the preciousness of your child with only words... Modesty is to acknowledge other people's existence and value them as they are...Respecting those who deserve your respect, be kind to the people who deserve your kindness...and to know your correct position in the world... That is modesty...Love grows on modesty... Hence, check how much modesty you have within... If you see it grow in you, your soul grows as well...

K: How should we understand those who practice self-training in search of the Truth and maturity of their souls, especially those who seek various meditation or breathing techniques and pursue super-natural abilities?

W: (in a very firm and strong tone) ...Many are chasing after illusions... All who are persuaded by the various techniques will practice them for self-satisfaction... Ten thousand out of ten thousand, and a hundred million out of a hundred million of such people practice for self-satisfaction... Only a handful out of uncountable numbers of people might go forward to the true growth of their souls... When a soul's growth reaches a certain level, it is no longer concerned with its own growth... The soul, then, turn its attention to the growth of those around it... Yet, unfortunately, people are contented only when seeing themselves change in various ways... That is only a first step... Moreover, when people keep practicing for self-satisfaction... the danger for themselves will keep growing as well... He will turn himself into a croaking frog... Please instruct me to 'go deeper'...

At his request, I repeated the instruction to deepen his hypnotic state and proceeded again. It may appear as if Won himself perceived that his state was too shallow to receive the message, but judging from the fact that he chooses the instruction he needs, according to his condition and 'orders' me to give him the needed words, I believe it is the Voice who 'orders' me through Won's mouth. They may have thought Won needed to go deeper into his hypnotic state to better receive and relay their messages. When such orders were given to me in previous sessions, such as - 'sink heavier', 'go deeper', 'instruct me to go into the Third Room', Won's voice always changed to the solemn tone of the Voices. And the words were more in the manner of authoritative orders than kindly requests.

W: ...What can draw out the spiritual vibration in us is love and modesty... Through modesty, we can love... and when love becomes our foundation, sacrifice can be achieved... but, to confirm your love through self-sacrifice is an elementary level... Love through modesty... and sacrifice through love to help many to reach their goodness... and when such a process becomes your true delight, you are in tune with the vibration of the Universe...When Jesus came to earth, many Pharisees thought they became elephants by obeying the laws of their religion and observing the God's commandments... They thought they were elephants... They croaked loudly and rolled their dung... But, what happened? ...When the man of modesty and love appeared among them, their false images crumbled, and they were embarrassed before him ...Love and modesty is the reality of everything... It is the ultimate goal of the Truth... It is the Truth itself... Modesty is the field, and Love is the fruit... Which is more important between the two? ...The fruit, of course, is more important... But, how can you expect the fruit without the field for the tree to root? ...Many deride the sound of frogs, saying, 'Why are they so loud?' ...but they do not realize that the sound of their derisive laughter is also a croaking... When you remove the froth of your soul, you will be able to listen to your own croaking... You will be able to see the empty things you have been rolling to make them appear big... You have to detach yourself from such activities... You must tender the ground of your existence to grow the fruit of the Truth in you... Without accomplishing such tasks first, you cannot practice true love... You are unable to love others' souls, and you also can not vibrate or resonate with them... The one who is truly humble and loving has no other choice but to appear weak and inferior, because he removes his hypocrisy, pretense and false images... Not a proud mask to show people remain... But, they are the ones who are truly strong...

As the vibration of the Universe and the Truth are in their hearts, with the power of those, they will sweep away the false images and the products of hypocrisy people have constructed... In the coming age, people who subject themselves to humiliation by removing their pretenses will embarrass the people who made themselves high and noble by hiding their faults... (in a strong tone) ...So far, the hypocrisy and false images of people may have kept them noble ...But, the time will change... (as if lamenting)... Truly, the time will come when one who is really humble will become a leader... Through humility, not self-degradation, he will console and support many souls and share spiritual growth with them... (after a brief pause)... There is a secret in a drink bottle...An alcoholic drink changes its own nature to make people exhilarated...Yes, we must fill ourselves with the yeast called 'Love' ...When we are filled and ferment with love, our forms and taste will change into new ones... to exhilarate people... Those who walk ahead of their time must ferment themselves first...We should become like a drink... A person who ferments himself with love, and makes others exhilarated... Yet, we must understand that good grapes make good wine, whereas bad grapes make low quality wine... Cultivate well your grape orchard...Please, produce a fragrant wine... (after a short silence) ...I see a rice bin... I see a rice worm eating the rice in it... I am told, the rice worm in the bin has a limited life span... I don't understand the meaning of this message...

K: Can I ask questions?

W: Yes...

K: Why is the population on earth keeps growing?

W: ...There have to be more new experiences ...One soul shall acquire many different experiences through various bodies, and new realizations will happen in this way... When the population reaches a certain level, it will reorganize itself... When the new era opens, the population will shrink to less than one tenth of the current size... A soul will learn new things in various bodies, and the evil will become more evil... and the virtuous will become more virtuous...

K: Is it possible for a soul to occupy various bodies? Are there such cases now?

W: Yes...

K: Will calamity and plague reduce the size of the population to less than one tenth of what we have now?

W: ...I hope... It would not be that way...

K: Do you mean the method of population reduction will depend on the actions and realization of people?

W: ...It is like having to decide whether to paint water color or oil upon the sketch or design already on the canvas... The sketch is drawn by the God, but the painting upon it can be decided by people...

K: When it happens, where do the souls without human body go? Without reaching the realization of themselves, where do they go?

W: ...They will come together...

K: Into a large congregation?

W: Yes... they will initially come together into one... Coming together does not mean all the souls will combine into a mass... It means they will forget their original states... and they will be sent off to somewhere... And I see the images of judgment and a courthouse...

K: Each of them face judgment after being sent off?

W: Now, I have two images appearing at the same time in my mind, one is about the judgment, and the other's meaning is 'All souls will arrive at the Truth.' ...I don't know how to interpret this...

K: Will the souls grow even after the judgment and reach realization of themselves?

W: ...It is too grand a subject to be understood by human wisdom...

K: Relax and rest... Do not try to explain it correctly... just relax... Do you hear the Voices?

W: ...I hear beautiful music...The Voices will not speak any more...

K: Shall we stop here today?

W: Yes...

Ninth session also taught me many things. After finishing his life as a foreman in Egypt, I heard, for the first time, about a place which we may call 'Hell'. Although Masai warrior Undihte had spent some time in a village after his death, repenting the killing of one of his fellow villager while alive, Won described the place as more like a 'purgatory' or a 'limbo'. Unlike the killing of a villager in a spell of blinding rage, the Egyptian foreman lived an intentionally malevolent life. Won told me that he only wished to escape from the hellish place because of the formidable pain he suffered there. He suffered much more pain than he inflicted upon others while living. McConell, the Scottish shepherd - We met him in the third regression- also stated that he realized his wrongdoings in a dark place after death. Though he suffered from the realization of his faults, he didn't experience such a vivid pain as this. These different memories may suggest a fact that our actions in a lifetime influence the after-death experiences to appear in many ways.

In other words those black and white ideas of heaven or hell. The past life regressions with other patients of mine also confirmed this supposition. When a life, though laden with misdeeds and mistakes that cannot be called evil was ended, all the patients recalled the memory of comfort and peace. Even though the death itself was very painful and tragic, comfort and peace were experienced beyond the moment of death. After that, most of the patients recalled they were guided by a light to somewhere beyond this world. Their report usually ends at this point. In Won's case also, the only detailed experience he recalled of the realm between lives is the account of Undihte. If I tried harder to explore more deeply into the after-life experiences, I am sure he could have recalled more memories of the realm. In all sessions so far with Won, I did not push him into any specific direction because I had decided in my mind, from the first session, only to follow whatever course Won takes. If we were to suppose that the place where he felt unbearable pain was 'hell', there must be an end to the suffering in hell because Won's soul was reborn to this world after the experience. The degree of suffering we get after death may reflect the life we finished, and the suffering seems to be an inevitable experience in the growth and progress of souls.

Furthermore, we should understand that the pain and suffering after death is not a revenge or repayment for his wrongdoing in life. Its purpose is to awaken the soul from the darkness it was in, and to make it realize the goal of its progress. The reality of hell may be only a state, in which extreme pain is given to purify its wrongdoing and to let it realize what pain he had given to others while alive. I thought, it was interesting that one of his superiors in office in this life was the man who stabbed Won to revenge for Won's taking away of his assets and daughter. The man have been harassing Won whenever he had a chance to do so.

A common pattern of transmigration is that the souls of good relationships in past lives tend to have friendly relationships in the present life, whereas, souls in hostile relationships will have similar adverse relationships in this life. For example, a loving husband and wife, or good parents and children, tend to meet again in good relationships, while those who had been enemies will meet in hostile relationships. I have seen this pattern more frequently than the opposite in many cases of patients including Won. The relationship between Won and the superior in the office is an example of this pattern. But, Won's hatred toward the superior has diminished significantly after he realized the evil things he had done on the man in the past life. He tells me that he feels peaceful at work since he understood the superior's attitude toward him through past life regression. Won accepts the fact that he has much debt to repay the man. The explanation on the failures of revolutions and social reformations is also very persuasive. People's inability to overcome their fundamental selfishness is the real reason why such movements can change only the surface of the society, never resolving the basic problems of the society. I can sympathize more with this simple explanation than the more complex ones offered by sociologists and politicians. Who would oppose to the idea that we can prevent and resolve most injustice and inequality of our society, the products of our selfishness, by sharing altruism? Although it may sound too simple a logic to our ears, I don't doubt this to be the most truthful answer.

Without having love and altruism, no matter how complex and well thought out theories we have, cannot give us true answer. 'Icarus' is a figure in Greek mythology. He soared into the sky with wax attached artificial wings. When he got too close to the sun, the wax which held together the wings melted, and he fell down to his death. This story metaphorically illustrates the emptiness of our various endeavors which relies on logic and intelligence alone, without basic knowledge of our foundation of existence. There are many types of self-discipline studies and meditation techniques that have nothing to do with true realization of the Truth. Achievements in such areas usually lead us to self-satisfactory contentment and overconfidence in our ability that derail us from the modest and serious quest to find out 'Who am I, and where have I come from?'. Self-justification becomes necessary to cover up this derailment. Numerous cult religions, hypocritical faiths and the people who claim to know about souls, without having love in them fall into this category. The metaphors of elephant, frog and dung-beetle describe the general tendency of the world today. They are a warning to the world of exaggerated self-advertisement, the world of wasting many times more than we have and the people who talk much more than they know. The metaphors also teach us to strive to build up the capacity of our souls to find the Truth in this overblown world. Among the readers, I am sure some will feel uneasy about religious, particularly Christian, overtone of the message regarding the maturity of soul, love and humility. But, the Voices never supported or encouraged any particular religion, on the contrary, they emphasized that any religion with no practice of its teachings is hypocrisy and no more than a self-adornment. To my view, the message from the Voices is full of teachings applicable to all of us, regardless of religious differences and cultures. Although the words, 'Jesus' and 'God' often mentioned in the message, they also talk about Buddha as well. Perhaps the Voices are using Christian terms to help our understanding because Won happens to be a Christian in his current life. If he had been a Buddhist, I am sure the Voices would have used Buddhist terms more often. The explanation about population increase was rather different from the one given by Edgar Cayce. He claimed that the population increase on earth is being caused by the return of the souls of those who had lived in ancient Atlantis. There has been a theory in parapsychology that says a soul can occupy more than one body at the same time. Although we don't know the exact mechanism of these phenomena, the Voices confirmed this can be true in some cases, and such cases also have the purpose, 'To learn from various experiences'. In time, I am sure we will understand better the subjects of 'reduction of population'. 'Gathering of souls', 'judgment and arriving at the Truth'.

CHAPTER 11

The Tenth Meeting:

The Meaning of Suffering, True Mental Training, Peace and War, Prophecies and Teachings.

(Won did not regress into past life memories. After reaching deep relaxation in a short time, he immediately connected to the Voices).

W: ...You should be content with your current life... but, you should not become idle in it... When you become idle in your limited situations, there will be no more spiritual growth and development... Regarding the growth of a soul... the Voices show me a rough and coarse skin... what the skin represents is... In the severe cold and strong wind, in rainstorms, our skin turns into a coarse and unattractive one... but it becomes strong and tough... by the same principle, our appearance may turn ugly after suffering hardship... it becomes more resilient and strong... Hence, various hardships we experience in life are like training programs given to us by the God...

K: Do you see anything around you?

W: ...I see a cabbage... The cabbage has a tendency to spread wide, but farmers tie it up with rope... What worth would a life have if everyone in this world live the selfish way they desire? ... When the God ropes you up, you may feel confined tight... But you will develop your worthiness as a product of that binding... Live a life in which you can enjoy the confinements the life presents to you... Such confinements act as focal strong points of your energy when you grow spiritually... All the hardships you face in your pursuit of really virtuous life are the God's blessings. Your soul will grow when you accept them as blessings... Your life will flourish the most in them... Although your suffering seems endless and the exit from them is never in sight, in the humble acceptance and endurance, your being will be gradually filled with growth and fulfillment... You will become like the cabbage with dense and tender leaves inside... You may ask why evil ones revel in the material abundance and monetary success... Let me ask you a question, 'Is it a blessed life which is filled with money, fame and comfort?'...(in a slow and strong tone) ...It is not so... You can have material goods and comfort only for a limited time... and they will rot away eventually... Memory of those days will bring you only the more bitterness... but, those who seem to be abandoned by God... those who appreciate their confinement and deficiency in honest pursuit of truthful life... will harvest their souls' growth and maturity...Physical limits and mental limits, the principle of overcoming limits is the same in either case... Consider this... Don't you build up your immunity by injecting vaccine into your own body? ...Small pain is the vaccine for a larger one... You can build the antibody to overcome the difficulties this way...The message ends here.

K: Relax and rest...

W: I hear the words...'The empty things of the world' and I see a frowning face of Sungchul (a famous Korean Buddhist monk who died a few years ago) ...The reason for his frowning... the Voices tell me, it is the state of his soul.

K: What kind of a person was he?

W: ...He worked hard to expand the realm of human mind... Yet, he is now in a new state of remorse... because; he faced another limit after his death... Eventually, he has realized the lamentable weakness of human ability and power...

K: Does he feel disappointed in the realm of spirits?

W: ...He feels disappointed in his own life...

K: Is it because he lacked love?

W: ...(in a pitying tone) ...You can say that, but, the more important thing is, he had forgotten his own existence, the foundation of his existence... He had only focused on his spiritual growth without exploring the origin and the foundation of his existence... As a result, he has found that his soul is unstable, as if it were a house built on sand...He realized this only after death... His soul is not at peace... We must not forget our foundation of existence in all of our spiritual practice and disciplines...We must make harmony with the God... and we must achieve this harmony from where we stand now... When we forget this, all our efforts and labor will become meaningless...

It will only make us more exhausted... In the long history of human society, numerous philosophers have taught people many philosophies... But, many of their souls suffered because they themselves were not able to understand the very foundation of their existence... This is like building a house without laying a solid foundation... The house will crumble down by a small shaking of the earth...Thus, we must make firm the foundation of our existence, and this should be the starting point of spiritual growth and development... People must realize that they can wish to love... but, they are not able to give true love... They are not the center of the Universe...They are only a part of it... The most important realization people can achieve is knowing where they ought to be... not enlarging their territory of existence... This will help make true harmony...

K: Relax and rest... Proceed only when you see or hear meaningful things...

W: ...The Voices are concerned about the campaign against leukemia which is in progress... They say, 'The campaign leads people by appealing to people's impulsive emotions instead of bringing out sincere love from them. Falsehood and pretense run deep in this campaign because it lacks true love... The campaign will only become another way to glorify certain people's name... The campaign has already strayed away from the realm of love to the realm of self-obsession... There are many movements and campaigns that intend to help suffering people... but they lose vitality when led only by general flow and emotions, not with true love... Most campaigns lose strength during their process because they tend to just follow the trend without true love as a motive in them... When the once heated emotions cool down, people will return to their original un-loving state... Another reason why we don't like such movements is, there are people behind the campaign who will get real benefit from the campaign... and they try to empower it... Owners of clinics expect an increase in their profits by performing many more bone marrow transplant operations, and the TV broadcasting companies want to imprint righteous images of them in the mind of audience... This is only an example...

...Message stops here... (after a brief pause) ...True love and good doings are not to decorate them with beautiful images ...To let your good deed be known and to enjoy such publicity... is an act of following false images... True reason for not letting others know your good deeds is to harvest the true fruit of them, they help your soul to grow and mature... to enable you to advance toward the God...Good deeds to enjoy fame and moralistic satisfaction do not have anything to do with your spiritual growth... They do not focus your soul's energy to grow... They are not good deeds at all... There is no love and humility in them... They don't last as patience is lacking in them... Many work hard to beautify themselves with attractive images and show off... But, it is all in vain... Useless efforts they are... Do not show off... Practice concealment... Do not expect rewards... Be content with the fact that your soul progress and evolve toward the original form which was given by the God... It is the biggest reward you get... the biggest compensation for your endeavor... This is the way you come closer to the God... Imprinting his image and form within your soul, becoming more like him... place yourself where you belong as a part of him... to fulfill the ultimate purpose of your existence... Virtuous looking life with nothing to do with spiritual growth only adds suffering to your days... it leaves only moral pleasure... You must do away with such a life... (after a short silence)... A common fallacy which many spiritual leaders in Korea are committing is... They believe their ability is a product of their own talents... and, instead of serving people in many nations with humility; they are becoming intoxicated by their power... You must serve... Numerous countries confirmed their power by dominating the world in the past... Now is the time for this country to confirm its authority by serving other countries... An authority, born from love and respect... more people and volunteers must strive for this...It doesn't mean they actually achieve some good results...but they create the atmosphere and the spiritual resonance for them...(in a convinced, strong tone)... The day when the evil forces will fall is not far away... I see a frowning face of a being that you can call Satan... Gradually, the innocent ones, naive ones will become leaders... Domination by force will come to an end...although it doesn't disappear completely... A new form of confrontation... The message stops here... (after resting a while) ...I see signs of a new war, airplanes are taking off from a carrier...Where can this be?... It is Middle East... North Africa... How many tears have we truly shed for the victims of war... The Voices are deeply grieving such calamities... The history of war since the beginning of human existence... We must yearn for the time of peace after the end of our war era... We must embrace, deep inside our heart, the souls of those who suffer from war... (in a very agonizing tone)... We must pray with the shuddering souls that are oppressed by fear, starvation and despair. We must resonate our souls with theirs... When we enjoy our comfort, those on the other side are frightened and famished in the ruins of war...In our own suffering, our souls must open eyes to them... We must pray as hard as they might in the ruins, to have their sufferings be lifted... In prayers, the Voices are heart-broken...

(Sighs and moans in agony for about a minute)... I now see a thirteen year girl in the middle of a ruined city... She has a stupefied and dazed look... She has lost her parents... She is in a refugee camp... No one takes care of her... She must grow by herself... (In a very loud and strong tone)... We must resonate our souls and connect our hearts to her blood vessels... with love, through love... I must have the incurably damaged heart of hers... We must send our love to those far away, even though we cannot see them... Sending them foods, material goods and organizing systems to help them is not enough... The day of peace will come to this world, only when people truly seek it from the bottom of their hearts and souls... We must seek it from the God... We must tune our vibrations to the frequency of the Universe... and by drawing on the power of the Universe, we must destroy the war, fear and starvation that rampage this world... They should be put to the torch so that they will never rise again... Burn them with the torch of love... Love, the most powerful energy in the Universe... We must rule all the forces that work against the current of the Universe... With the heart that seeks peace, with the heart that loves souls... We must carry on this task... The message ends here.

The magnitude of the emotional energy that poured out with these words was overwhelming. Compassion and sadness were dissolved in every word he spoke, and the sighing and lamenting from the deep of his heart vibrated in his shuddering voice. Overwhelmed, I could only watch the heartbreaking resonance of his soul. It was an expression of the true love and compassion toward those who suffer. He also spoke in a very strong and confident tone, emphasizing each word, when talking about the evil forces. When the message ended, I told him to rest a while, and after a short pause, he started to deliver another teaching.

W: A new teaching is being given by showing me an image of soybean being ground under a millstone to become tofu...

K: Listen to it.

W: ...When we try to serve others, it is difficult for you to benefit them directly, because we are like hardened soybeans over time... We must soak ourselves in water, and grind ourselves under the millstone to decompose our shape and hardness... then, we can become soft tofu to be eaten by many... This is the way how we serve others... The sufferings of many good, innocent people are this tofu making grinding process... They must go through this process of soaking their rigid hearts, grinding off their peels and breaking their original shapes... Without this process, they can't get into others... They cannot become flexible enough... If you go through much suffering, if you go through the pain like you are being grind between a set of millstone even though you have decided to live a truthful life...Consider your pain as the grinding off of unbecoming parts in you... Does the chemical composition of soybean change because it is ground between millstones? ...Of course not... Only physical properties that make it difficult for people to digest soybean change... Yes... We must grind off, between millstones, our edges and corners without losing the noble form which the God bestowed on us... We must grind and purify ourselves through life's ordeals and hardship this world presents us... They say I should stop here today...

Pain and hardship, the Voices stated, are trainings given to us by the God for our souls to mature. They also said that, to stay inside the present happiness is to stop our growth and forgoing lessons to learn. The message about the high Buddhist priest who died a few years ago was rather surprising, because what the Voices told us was totally different from the popular belief that he had been an 'enlightened' one. But, I think I can understand what the Voices told us. It is always possible for anyone to forget the foundation of his existence and humble beginning when he submerges himself in ascetic practices of many forms to achieve personal abilities to a heroic degree. Personal progress can become an obsession as well. Although his life-long exertion while alive may become a great helping karma in his next reincarnation, the Voices pointed out that he had many regrets as well. They also said that practices to attain supernatural or psycho-kinetic power are only for self-satisfaction and overconfidence, and have nothing to do with spiritual growth. The Voices emphasized again that we can never reach the Truth, however hard we may practice, while forgetting the basis of our existence. Practicing good deeds without advertising, the warning to the various campaigns and movements are good lessons to remember. The Voices seemed to give rather optimistic forecast for the future of Korea. As mentioned in previous sessions, they claimed Korea has an important role in the future world. I can only describe Won's overwhelming outburst of emotions, when appealing for the resonance of our souls and compassion toward those who are suffering the atrocities of war, as an expression of the God's true love for humanity.

CHAPTER 12

[Below is another message given to us in a different session than the ten sessions introduced above. I have decided to include it because its contents are related to those of other messages: Awe of life, Witch hunt, the true and the false].

W: …I hear the Voices…

K: Listen to them.

W: (in a deep and heavy tone) …It is not the good results of your action that determines where you must go… It is a motive like 'I want to live a good life' that triggered your good actions… Destruction of life is the gravest action of terror… The God wishes to preserve life… Other manners of death than natural ones are all crimes… sinful actions… Do not intend to kill the 'bad' insects only because they irritate us… As every life form has its reason to exist, death is possible only when the reason of its existence disappear… Thus, suicide is not right… and we should not kill at will even a bug… We should not destroy the bug's life because it is an expression of the essential existence of a being, and the reason of existence of the bug's individual life is not fulfilled yet… (in a dark and sad tone)… Now, the ongoing destruction of environments by current materialistic civilization is a terrible process which destroys the order of life and will bring horrible consequences… The movement to prevent the destruction of environment has its flaws, because it aims to protect environment to have better places for people to live in… But, the true protection of environment should start from the awe of life… The destruction of countless individual lives that follows the destruction of environment... Only when we have a sincere desire to protect those lives, true protection of environment is possible... Many people want to protect environment to have more, to enjoy safer life themselves... But, it is a selfish behavior... Environmental protection movement should evolve to 'Respect for Life' movement... What is really important is our respect for each individual life and the right of the life to choose the way how to live... When we obey and follow the law and order of life, we can become one with the nature... Humanity will survive only when you accomplish this... The first step toward the Truth is possible when you understand this... The journey to the Truth begins with the 'Respect for life'... Disregard of the dignity of individual life leads to disconnection and destruction of relationships... damaged relationships heal only when you respect the individual life of the object... the Message ends here.

K: Relax and rest...

W: ...I see a shoehorn... It is a tool to help people to put on shoes... One who would help others should have clear identity of oneself... The meaning of the metaphor of the shoehorn is this... Ask yourself repeatedly, 'Why I exist here? Why do I have to live?, What shall I live for?' ...When the answers to these questions solidify inside of you, you will be able to give real help... One who forgets life is the one who throws life away... We need to cherish life...

W: The Voices are talking about 'Witch hunt'...'why did it start? Because the ruling class at the time was not able to control the people with new ideas effectively... The 'witch hunt' was a product of their struggle for self-defense.

...Now, you (me) can become victims of 'witch hunts'... Although witches never existed, witch hunts can happen even now... When people of the establishment lack self confidence in their authority, they try to show their power to public and secure their position and privilege through 'witch hunts'... Many arguments of heresy, legal prosecution and debates of legitimacy in many sectors of modern society are also other forms of witch hunt... One who judge others must have love, judging others without love will bring the judgment upon the one who judges... (in a very strong tone)... Therefore, you should not be swayed by the people who stir public to go against you... They are the ones who hide behind their social establishment, but they lack objective knowledge and judgment... (in a stronger voice)... Secure your territory more firmly when witch hunt gets ferocious...Have conviction in your mission of 'Love and the Truth' you have... You can have freedom to laugh at witch hunt... The Truth grows in denigration and disparagement... The Truth that is not denigrated and hated becomes a 'compromise'... I hear the word 'Inshallah'... Let the Truth take care of your life... Remember the words, 'Truth will set you free.' ...You are a man who has courage to protect the Truth... But, you must practice more to lower yourself before the God... Still, your self-consciousness is too strong... You should possess more humility before the God... Not before men... Practice it in your daily life... Good manners are not humility... As we told you before, humility is accepting other beings' existential value as it is... The message ends here..

K: Rest and relax as much as you need... (after resting for a minute)

W: ...Food shortage will become serious in the future... I see a boy in Africa moaning under the burning sun... The problem is not in the production of foods, it is in the distribution... There is a possibility of breakdown in the system of distribution... it will cause many conflicts... In the future, many conflicts will be between a nation and a business corporate... Some wars will be triggered by business people... And the time of suffering for many clerics will come...

K: Why will the clerics suffer?

W: ...Many of them will take the road to compromise... They will serve in the new set of values, and no small number of them will lose their lives...

K: Will there be a religious persecution?

W: Yes... especially, the Christians will suffer the most...

K: Is it also a process to improve the world from materialism?

W: (after a brief pause) ...In the future, clerics will be divided into two groups, one will accept compromise and another will not ...This division will be most distinct in Christians... Many religions will attempt to unite with others... But, the Christians will be the most intransigent to do so... On the surface, this unifying movement will appear to bring more peace... but, internally, it will distance religions from the Truth more... Thus, the people who compromise will take the path to the fall, and their souls will suffer... and the ones who don't compromise will suffer physical and material pains... Anyway, the authority of clerics will diminish like that of the Shaman's did long ago... (in a strong tone)... But, the ones who persevere to the end will have their share of the Truth ...I see a squid and an octopus...

K: What do they mean?

W: The way they take nutrition from other animals... squeezing other animal's body to death and absorb the body fluids...The way they immobilize the victim with their legs...The Voices tell us to escape from the suction force of tradition... To escape from traditional viewpoints does not mean to ignore traditions... It means that there is a need to reinterpret the real value of traditions... The future will become extremely confusing... it is a darkness before the arrival of the light...The message ends here.

K: Will you tell me about Shamans?

W: (after a pause)... I see dirty images... They are untidy... It is better not to have them in the world... But, they are useful in utilizing evil spirits... They have no love, no humility... and they have no desire to seek the Truth... They are used only in seducing people...

K: Are souls of dead people permitted to roam the world without going to spirit world?

W: ...It is not permitted in strict sense... But, they can choose... When they choose not to go, they suffer greater pain...

K: You mean, in time, all of them must go?

W: ...Unless, they will not be able to endure the increasing suffering and pain that accompany their decision to stay... It is a great pain not to go where they belong... The Voices want you not to pay much attention to shamans...

K: Is it because they are false?

W: Yes... the interest in wandering spirits and the life after death may distract your attention from more important truths... In time, you will know all the things you want... The most important thing is to cherish the truth, and let it show in your daily life... make it the frame of yourself, and make it the frame of your life... Too much curiosity will distract your focus from the truth, and you will lose the direction... (in a strong tone)... You will know the good when you focus on the evil... When you focus on the good, you will automatically understand the evil... But, when you know the good by focusing on the evil... You will not have the courage to do the good... And, when you know the evil by focusing on the good, you don't have to fight the evil...the evil will crumble by itself...You should remember this as you are a wise man... Look at the root of a big tree... trunk stretches out from it, and branches spread out from the trunk, and leaves will come out from the branches... Yes... the root, trunk, branch and the leaves...they all are components of a tree... But, not all the components are the same... The roots will always exist as long as the tree lives... branches can dry up, and the leaves will invariably fall off... At times, cocoon of a worm or a spider web clings to the leaves... Who will call the cocoon and spider web a tree? ...Who will call the withered leaves a tree?

...Are the leaves not a tree... They are a part of the tree... But, withered leaves are not... What decides whether it is a tree or not... The presence of life-force or death is the determining point... What is the truth and what is not... If there is life, it is the truth, and if there is no life-force, it is not... The question about stray spirits and shamans is like asking whether a spider web or a cocoon on the leaves of a tree is also a part of the tree... Now, you know the standard... The truth has life in it because it has love... if you want to know about a tree, look at the actions of life in it... Thus, you don't need to pay attention to dead or dried up things... The message ends here.

K: Rest and relax...

W: (after a brief rest)... It is possible to have a small body like a shrimp but have eyes that can look all over the ocean... And have a big body like a whale but have eyes that can see only small area in front... There are great looking people who actually don't know where to go, and there are shabby and stupid looking people who have wisdom in them... Many saints are hidden among the shabby and poor looking people who are now living in the world... They have sympathy for the Earth and the Universe... and endeavor to maintain such energy... sees a sprinter... When he is running at full speed on spikes, his body leans forward very much... Untrained people cannot run on spikes like a sprinter... But, the spikes are a good support to a sprinter... Likewise, when the same truth is given, it becomes a good tool to the prepared ones for their progress... But, as it becomes a burden to the unprepared ones, they throw it away and trample upon it... So, you should not throw your pearls before the pigs...Enlarge your bowl for the truth...Make your life a big bowl which can contain the truth more and more everyday...

I have not yet heard about environment protection movements that focus on the 'Awe of life'. But, the Voices warned about the countless lives that are being killed by the destruction of their habitats. To become one with the nature, we should understand the dignity and value of each and every individual life first, they advised. The messages regarding the true nature of witch hunt, the worry about the instability of future world, and the essence of shamans and the stray spirits, are all subjects we need to think about.

The Voices and Medium Channeling

You have so far read the transcript of the eleven hypnotic Past-Life Regression sessions of my patient Won. I am sure the readers' feelings and reactions to the text will be different, according to the cultural and religious background of each person. I, myself, am still unable to grasp the full meaning of this encounter with Won. Although my intention was to do the hypnotic therapies on him to improve his specific discomforts, the sessions turned out to be much different from what I expected. We were to be told various messages about many important subjects of life from mysterious spiritual entities - I decided to call them 'The Voices'. Their message consistently emphasized the value of love, sacrifice, patience and humility and told us some secrets of politicians of the past and present and prophecies regarding the future world. The Voices even encouraged us to help spread these messages far and wide, to enable people to prepare themselves for the future. Some of you might doubt the authenticity of the transcript of sessions with Won. But, if you think that I and Won conspired to fabricate the messages, it would be a nice compliment to us because it means we are exceedingly capable persons. We are simply not enlightened enough to make up such profound teachings of the Voices. Furthermore, it does not make much sense to fabricate false stories to spread the message of love and sacrifice. The reason why the Voices gave us the future prophecies is perhaps to add authority and authenticity to the messages, and to attract more people to listen to the messages to help them start the journey to spiritual self-realization.

The sessions with Won can be called 'Medium Channeling'. It is a scientifically controversial phenomenon. But, the examples of trance mediumship and messages delivered in this fashion are many from the ancient times in all cultures. Some of them are very well known to us, oracles in Greek mythology, prophesies in Bible, claims of the communication with spirits by mediums and shamans can be classified as 'medium channeling'. To be defined as a 'medium channeling', information and messages delivered should come from scientifically unexplainable sources or presumed spiritual entities through unknown mechanism, and the contents should be beyond the medium's education, experiences and cultural background. Although modern psychiatry does not openly accept the possibility of 'medium channeling' by spirits in trance state of a medium, it acknowledges the existence of many forms of unexplainable spiritual phenomena in human experiences. Most mediums have high susceptibility of hypnotic trance and are highly sensitive to spiritual or super-natural phenomena. My patient Won also showed these characteristics. The most famous medium of modern times must be Edgar Cayce of Virginia, USA. In hypnotic trance, he diagnosed and suggested successful remedies to the medical problems of thousands of people he never met, although he was not highly educated man and had no conscious knowledge of medicine. He gave more than 2,500 life-readings; in them he traced past lives of people and helped them to solve their current problems by understanding the roots of them in the past lives. American psychiatrist Brian Weiss called, in his book 'Many lives, Many masters', the mysterious spiritual beings 'Masters' that delivered messages similar to ours in hypnotic sessions with his patient Catherine. I also think 'The Voices' are highly developed spiritual entities, but I decided to call them simply 'The Voices' than other fancy name. They told us they are being called as 'holy spirits' in Christian religions and 'Buddha's mind' in Buddhism. In whatever name they may be called, I believe they are 'Transcendental and spiritual beings with intention to help humanity'.

The world today is in deep trouble. Traditional authorities are losing power rapidly over people and many ailments of materialism are spreading all over the world to cause large scale destruction and distortion in environments and climate. Corrupt politicians and business cartels are ignoring the dire warnings of climate cataclysm from various science fields to pursue only money and influence. The future of the world will fall into darkness unless we change the course of the present world. The messages from the Voices repeatedly emphasized love toward life and soul, sacrifice, patience and spiritual growth of us, as keys to solve the problems of the world. I never thought about publishing the messages of the Voices until I finished the fifth session with Won. But, as the sessions with Won progresses, I started to realize, these moving messages of hope were not meant only for me and Won.

About Mr. Jongjin Won – my patient and channeling medium

I got to know more about this young man as the sessions of past-life regression and Channeling with him progress. He is very considerate and kind to others and appeared more mature than his age of twenty-six. He is an intuitive person with composure and stable attitude. He always reflects on his words, thoughts and actions, and gives off soothing impression with his modest demeanor. The fact that he had to become the man of the house very early in his age due to his father's untimely death, probably contributed to his maturity. According to the retrieved memories of his past lives, he had lived a few lives as an ascetic. I believe these experiences as an ascetic must have left numerous traces in his present personality. After graduating from college, he moved from one employment to another, suffering frustrations, self-doubt and depression. He was trying to find a security of mind as a Christian at the end of his soul searching wandering, but unable to find answers for the ultimate issues of life, he got interested in the concepts of reincarnation and transmigration because he thought them very logical explanations to many puzzles of life. He chose to visit me after reading a self-report of a reporter about her own experience of hypnotic past-life regression session with me, in a news magazine. His future plan is to enroll in a graduate school of Christian theology to become a pastor of the protestant church. The Voices said he must be protected for now, because he has a mission in the future. After his recovering the memories of shared past-lives with me, we became closer in personal level. Considering his sincere attitude toward life, I think he will someday possess a high spiritual power if he sincerely prepares himself for some years. He used to have a few bad habits and flaws before he started hypnotic regression with me. When he encountered unfairness, he tended to overreact, sometimes with violent emotions.

And he used to have a self-righteous attitude which made him to look down slightly upon the same age group people. He also had a habit of over-eating when feeling frustrated. As he demanded perfection from himself and people around him, he got angry and depressed inside, when his high expectation was not met. Other than these problems, he also had his share of common anxieties of young man in employment, like, uncertain future and insecure position in the office.

However, since he started regression sessions with me, he is undergoing easily detectable changes in his life. First of all, he does not become violently furious anymore when facing unfairness and injustice, and has become readily forgiving and respecting people around him. His overeating habit has completely disappeared that he now can stop eating when feeling comfortable fullness. His perfectionism has changed into more relaxed, 'Well, it will be done in time.' attitude.

Although similar changes can be seen in people who started to believe in soul's growth and reincarnation, Won looks like a man who has achieved a great progress in his quest of the truth. He looks very secure, fully aware of his path, as if he were through all the wandering. I can see the determination in him that he wants to devote his life in complete earnestness to the quest of his soul. He also shows deep affection and trust towards me, and I feel as if he were my lost brother. After losing my only brother in this life, I might have attained a brother from one of my past-life. The Voices suggested me to treat Won like a young brother, a friend and a student, but I have already gotten more help from him. If he were to become a pastor, who would teach the truth not contaminated with sectarian religious dogmas, as the Voices suggested, I would like to help him in any way possible.

The changes I have gone through

Since I added the past-life regression to my other hypno-therapeutic techniques, significant changes have started to come over me. Although I had thought the concepts of Karma, transmigration and reincarnation as logical, they were valid only as theories in my head. But, as various patients improved and healed of their mental and physical symptoms through dramatic and moving experiences of the therapy, I have become more and more convinced of the validity of these ancient theories. Especially, the repeated encounter with the Voices in the sessions with Won has changed me deeply. I thought of myself as a bright and capable psychiatrist. I have been treating my patients with logical and impartial psychoanalytic theories and other principles of psychotherapy, as well as diverse medication, and I believe I have helped most of my patients. But, I often felt helpless when I meet the patients with unexplainable and unresponsive symptoms. Only temporary reliefs and superficial management of symptoms with most medication therapy depressed me as well. The limitation and insufficiency of materialism based neurology and psychiatry had made me, from long ago, to look into other cutting edge science fields than medicine everyday for the new answers to the mystery of human consciousness. Now, I am happy to know that the spiritual and supernatural aspects of human experiences can be explained by quantum physics and other emerging fields of science. The quantum computer like characteristics of human brain has also been discovered recently. The questions regarding the reality of human soul and the memories of past lives also can be logically explained by new discoveries and results of advanced experiments on human consciousness, and documented evidences of human consciousness functioning without brain activity are also accumulating in research of NDE (Near Death Experience). I believe we are now at the threshold of a drastic change of paradigm, as traditional materialism is losing ground and the new science of body-soul integration is replacing its place rapidly. The past-life regression therapy is just one example of how this emerging new knowledge can be utilized.

As I have witnessed many vivid emotions from my patients' past-life memories, death bed agonies and reflections of that life, spiritual awakening and realization of the connection between the past and the present problems, and the following improvement and disappearance of their symptoms. To my eyes, death simply does not occur to our souls, and I now fully accept the authenticity of the theories of reincarnation and transmigration, and I also have found some clues to solve my personal problems. I feel, I have become closer and kinder to my patients than before, and my emotional fluctuations and aggressiveness have decreased remarkably. Now, I realize more positive therapeutic results and deeper mutual understanding between me and the patient is possible when I try to tune myself to the vibration of the patient's emotion. When I look out the window of my clinic, each person who walks on the street below appears to me as one of my possible past or future self. And this thought brings me a smile and a heartwarming kindness towards them. Most patients who experience past-life regression report one or many of his close relations are the same person from other past lives. They recollect memories of past-lives shared by those around them. It means that we must have already met present family members, close friends and bitter enemies, hundreds or thousands years ago, in another life time, sometimes repeatedly. Roles and positions may change according to the necessity of a specific lifetime, but the continuing relationship of a group of people suggests, they are in the process of learning and growing through many life times to achieve the freedom from their Karmic circle, and the realization of their souls' true purpose. The biggest problem of modern psychiatry has been its blindness and unwillingness to look at the spiritual, supernatural experiences of people. The birth of 'Transpersonal

Psychiatry' in 1969 was possible by a bunch of frustrated, like I, psychiatrists and psychologists. Since then, the science about human consciousness is discovering many new aspects of human brain function and mind operation.

Still, the Transpersonal Psychiatry is not on the center stage of psychiatry, but I am sure, in the future, by the help of quantum physics, quantum biology and the research results of Near Death Experience, the existence of human soul and its survival of the death of physical body will be accepted as a serious subject of research and consideration of mainstream science.

About myself

Since my early childhood, I was deeply interested in the fundamental questions of life. From middle school days, I began my wandering to search for the answers to those questions. But, to my dismay, I was unable to find satisfying answers anywhere. All the books I read and the churches I attended with sincerity gave me no fulfilling answers. To my eyes at that age, all those with deep faith who entrusted their life completely to God were cowards who irresponsibly cling to more powerful being. And the theory of transmigration and reincarnation was the most ridiculous of all superstitions; because there could be no 'real self' if we were to have ever-changing bodies and identities. Thus, Buddhism, which teaches transmigration, was only a subdivision of superstition, and the love of God in Christianity also seemed like a total violence, because we get tossed into hell to suffer if we were not to follow God's words. To me, such a threat was no different from that of a street thug. I could only hope vaguely at the time that there would be more logical and convincing explanations to our life and the universe. When I was a second grader in the middle school, at age 14, I came across the book 'Interpretation of Dreams' by Sigmund Freud in one of the used bookstores I frequented. As I knew he was the founder of the theories of psychoanalysis, I opened the book. It was filled with small letters and difficult vocabularies written in old Chinese characters that seemed to hold some answers to the mysteries of life. I immersed myself in the book from that day, not because the content of the book made much sense to a middle school boy, but because Freud's sincere endeavor to explain human psyche with difficult concepts and words seemed so cool and intellectual to me.

When I finished reading this difficult book, I was happy with the intellectual gratification. Since then, I seriously began digging into difficult-looking books about variety of philosophy and theology during my high school and college years. But, I was unable to find the satisfactory answers to the basic questions of life. Every branch of philosophy and theology was unessential and partial to my view. All the philosophers seemed to be talking about small alleys while I was searching for an ocean. I have never been interested in pursuing the truth through ascetic self discipline or religion. The strong impression left by Freud's book made me wish to become a psychiatrist someday, and I vaguely felt that I would become able to find the truth by becoming one myself. However, at the time of graduation from medical school, I was disappointed in psychiatry. What I saw in the in-patient ward of psychiatry, during my one month long practice days, was a stagnant atmosphere of the doctors and nurses, and the patients who were under the heavy influence of medication. Not a patient was completely healed despite heavy medication and long talk therapies. Nonetheless, my path of the future was already chosen in my middle school days. When I had to choose the branch of medicine, of which I wanted to become a specialist, I consulted one of my senior who was a resident doctor of psychiatry in a general hospital, because I was disappointed in psychiatry. He said to me after listening to my dilemma, 'If you want to study very much, apply for Internal Medicine. And If you want to study much more than that, choose Psychiatry.' These words sealed my fate, and I have no regrets. His words inspired me to choose psychiatry as the main tool for my search for the answers to the mysteries of life. Since then, I have been learning so much from my patients. Every psychiatric patient is different. If there were a hundred patients suffering from depression, it means there are a hundred different types of depression to deal with. Psychiatrists must have sincere interest and affection for their patients, but interest and affection alone is not enough, they must have the ability to resolve the patients' problems as well. Although every doctor must continue to study new knowledge of medicine and science, but psychiatrists must not only study but also mature in their personality and spirituality. They must be more open minded than other doctors because they frequently have to deal with stranger symptoms and unexplainable phenomena.

Brief history of Past-Life Regression Therapy

Although the purpose of this book is not to discuss hypnosis or Past-Life Regression Therapy itself, a brief history of the therapy will be of help to most of the readers to understand better the contents of this book. Before 1960, there had been almost no report of past-life memory; and even if there have been any, the public paid little attention to it. Out of this scarcity, a book titled 'The search for Bridey Murphy' was published in 1956, This book described an incident about hypnotic past life regressions of a woman named Virginia Burns Tighe, from 1952 until 1953, by the author of the book, Morey Bernstein from Colorado. The regression work found a past life of Mrs. Tighe in Belfast, Ireland, in the 19th century. Skepticism and controversy arose not only in readers, the author himself was skeptical at the beginning, but, as the regressions repeated, he became convinced of the authenticity of the past life memories of Mrs. Tighe. Many detailed pieces of memory recovered were verified by documents and historians of Belfast, and Murphy's distinct accent of Irish slum language was impossible for Mrs. Tighe to have acquired or been taught by someone, prior to the regression, because no American entertainer ever used it. The book 'Children who remember their past lives – Twenty cases suggestive of reincarnation' was published by Dr. Ian Stevenson, in 1966. He was a psychiatrist and a pioneer in the research of reincarnation. He wrote massive two volume book,

'Reincarnation and Biology: A contribution to the Etiology of Birthmarks and Birth Defects' in 1997. More than 14 books and hundreds of papers about reincarnation were written by him. As all his works were based on very rigorous scientific verification methods, he is acknowledged as one of the most authoritative researchers in the field. In 1967, an English psychiatrist, Denys Kelsey published a book, named 'Many Lives' with Joan Grant who recalled her past life memories. Four books published in 1978, were very important in the history of past life regression therapy. They are 'Reliving Past Lives' by Helen Wambach, 'You have been here before', by Edith Fiore, 'Past Life Therapy' by Morris Netherton, 'Voices from Other Lives' by Thorwald Dethlefsen.

In the 1970s, the practice of this therapy was focused on its potential to relieve various unexplainable symptoms. But in the 1980s, the focus of interest shifted to human soul's pilgrimage and the meaning of life. The influence of new theories and discoveries of consciousness research and other advanced scientific fields including quantum physics and quantum biology, made some scientists, including medical doctors, to conclude that the 'ultimate being' of human existence is 'consciousness' and it survives death of the physical body. Towards the end of the 1980s, some scientists saw human body as 'Energy Fields' and tried to develop concept of medical treatment as a 'change in the energy'. Some of the influential books of this era are 'Recovery of the Soul' (1989), by Larry Dossey, 'Love, Medicine, and Miracles' (1988), by Bernie Siegel, and 'Quantum Healing' (1989), by Deepak Chopra. Other important books of the same era about Past-lives, written by psychiatrists, are 'Life between Life' (1986) by Joel Whitton, 'Many Lives, Many Masters '(1989), by Brian Weiss, 'Coming back' (1990), by Raymond Moody, 'Other Lives, Other Selves' (1987) by Roger Woolger, and 'Who were you before you were you?' (1990) by Garret Oppenheim. Since the introduction of the Past-life regression therapy in the 1960s, many psychologists and psychiatrists have dismissed it as fantasy, pseudo-memory or source-amnesia. The therapists who accepted this therapy in their practice were usually ridiculed and met with harsh criticism from their peers. But, reports of successful treatment of patients by the technique continued. In 1988, eighteen authoritative experts on memories in hypnosis published a book titled 'Hypnosis and Memory', after extensive research and case reviews of all the issues regarding memories in hypnosis including past life regression therapy. Some excerpts from the book are as follows. 'Reincarnation is a spiritual belief that meets our criterion of acceptability: Believing in it does no harm to other people.' 'The scientific method is probably too blunt a method to confirm or disconfirm the hypotheses of reincarnation or an afterlife. In the clinical situation there is usually no need to independently verify the truth or falsity of hypnotically elicited memories given the long-standing clinical belief that it can be just as effective to treat a person's fantasies of his or her past as it is to treat documented realities of that past. Moreover, data suggests that 'reincarnation therapy which depends upon a regression procedure may benefit a percentage of patients.' 'The Synopsis of Psychiatry' is one of the main textbooks of psychiatry for medical students and doctors worldwide. In the 1998 edition, Past-life regression therapy was included among newly introduced therapies of psychiatry. It was the first official acknowledgement of the therapy as an effective and legitimate tool for psychiatrists. In the 2000s, books and case reports of past-life memories are steadily increasing in volume and the authenticity of some of the cases were verified by evidences. Along with the testimonies of NDE (Near Death Experience), past life memories are strong evidence of the possibility of the survival of human consciousness after physical death.

Closing Words

It is unreasonable to live without knowing who we really are. It is like having no subject to an action. If I live without knowing why I live, it is the same as having no known purpose to my life. If I have no idea of the subject and the object of my life, I will not be able to live a meaningful life, as my existence here would be defined as an aimless wandering. To me, seeking the truth is to get the answers to these two questions of my existence.

The concepts of Transmigration and Karma, Past-Life and Reincarnation, Hypnosis and Subconscious Memory mentioned in this book, have their own complicated theories behind their names. The purpose of this book, however, is not to discuss the complexity of them, but to share many teachings and prophecies given by a mysterious source, which I called 'The Voices', during past-life regression sessions with one of my patients. When you open your heart and listen to the messages and prophecies in the dialogue shared here, I am sure many of you will feel the same way as I did. The Voices told us that the messages are blessings from God to prepare us for the time to come. Materialism has failed to deliver true contentment to humanity, because the true nature of humanity is not material, but spiritual. The realization that I am an everlasting being made of immortal soul often serves as a vital force to accept any difficult situation and to keep hope through it.

I have to be responsible for my actions, and need to understand that everyone around me came to earth to learn and grow as I did, and I have to help and love all people as myself. Following this simple and clear path is the only way to complete the truth of my life. The teachings of the Voices make us to ponder about the existence of a God and the essence of our being. When we believe that the meetings with our loved ones have continued through endless periods of time over many lifetimes, our love toward them will become even deeper, and when you understand those who trouble you have their own reasons embedded in the Karma between you and them, you will be able to overcome the difficulties in your relationship with them. As love and humility grow in us, our souls will grow and mature as well. Through this process, we will overcome the influence of negative Karma in our lives and tune ourselves to the frequency of love, the fundamental principle of the Universe. In the end, we will realize that we are the ones that God shares his life with, and death is only a process that leads to another beginning phase of life; there is no permanent parting, and all negative emotions and thoughts are only illusions… all the sufferings we go through in life is fertilizer and blessing for the growth of our soul…

END

About the Author

Youngwoo Kim, MD, is a specialist in transpersonal hypnotherapy and biofield therapy who introduced past-life regression therapy to Korea in 1995. Kim has run a Seoul-based clinic for thirty years, accumulating more than forty thousand hours of hypnotherapy sessions over the course of his career. His cutting-edge research into topics like Quantum Physics, Transpersonal Experiences, Spirit Possession, Multiple Personality Disorder and the connections between these subjects have set him apart from his peers. He is the founder and chairperson of the Korean Society of Transpersonal Psychiatry and a member of both the Korean Neuro-Psychiatry Association (KNPA) and the American Psychiatric Association (APA).